Women's Disclosure of Childhood Sexual Abuse Across the Life Course

Taking a narrative approach, this book explores the role of disclosure in sexual abuse recovery for women survivors of child sexual abuse.

Drawing on longitudinal research with sexual abuse therapists and de-identified cases drawn from her clinical practice, Pack emphasises the unique value of both a narrative and life course approach to the topic of sexual abuse recovery. The book explores the ages and stages of life as triggering new challenges to adapt to for adult women survivors, evoking the need to develop new ways of acting and being in the world. Conceptualising disclosure as a process that occurs in relationship with the person disclosed to, it highlights the importance of the quality of the relationship between the survivor and the person confided in and previous disclosure attempts. Further, the chapters outline individual, contextual and environmental factors that impede or facilitate disclosure, as well as different verbal and non-verbal forms that disclosure can take.

With a focus on the Australasian context, this book is a resourceful guide for mental health professionals and practitioners who work in the field of sexual abuse recovery, as well as those who work with women in refuge situations and other health and wellbeing services.

Margaret Pack is Associate Professor at Otago University of Wellington and counselling co-ordinator at Wellington Hospital, Wellington, New Zealand. She has ten years of experience as a specialist case manager in a national trauma centre in New Zealand and clinically supervises counsellors, social workers and mental health professionals.

Women's Disclosure of Childhood Sexual Abuse Across the Life Course

A Narrative Perspective

Margaret Pack

Routledge
Taylor & Francis Group
LONDON AND NEW YORK

Designed cover image: Photo of Woman of Words statue by artist Virginia King, New Zealand

First published 2025
by Routledge
4 Park Square, Milton Park, Abingdon, Oxon OX14 4RN

and by Routledge
605 Third Avenue, New York, NY 10158

Routledge is an imprint of the Taylor & Francis Group, an informa business

British Library Cataloguing-in-Publication Data
A catalogue record for this book is available from the British Library

ISBN: 978-1-032-66919-9 (hbk)
ISBN: 978-1-032-66915-1 (pbk)
ISBN: 978-1-032-66920-5 (ebk)

DOI: 10.4324/9781032669205

Typeset in Times New Roman
by Taylor & Francis Books

For Bob and Beryl

Contents

Illustrations

Figures

Tables

Acknowledgements

I wish to acknowledge my debt to the founding work of the following theorists for their original research on disclosure, including: Professor Ramona Alaggia, Professor Sarah Ullman, Dr Jewell Brazelton and Dr Rosaleen McElvaney.

I wish to thank also the founding theorists of the New Trauma Therapy who include: Drs Judith Herman, John Briere, Christine Courtois, and Constance Dallenburg; the founding work of the attachment theorists; and narrative theorists Michael White and David Epston, all of whose work I have found invaluable to refer back to as I was writing.

On a personal note, many friends and colleagues have contributed their time in helping me to write this book. I am particularly indebted to Anna Ormond and Michael Fauchelle, librarians at Otago University of Wellington, New Zealand, for undertaking literature searches for me and doing final reference checking. Thanks also to Justin Cargill, senior librarian of Victoria University of Wellington, New Zealand, for assisting me in the initial literature search that started my research for this book. A special note of thanks to Andrea Collins, of Te Whatu Ora, who formatted my diagrams expertly.

I also wish to thank my editorial assistants at Routledge, for their assistance and advice throughout the project.

On a personal note I wish to thank Robyn Pack, my sister, for caring for my wellbeing throughout the writing process. With such loyal and faithful support, all things seem possible.

Preface

As this book goes into production, I wish to explain the significance of the front cover and its relationship to the topic of disclosure by women survivors of childhood sexual abuse. The image on the book's cover is a photograph I took of the stainless-steel sculpture 'Woman of Words' by renowned sculptor Virginia King. This imposing figure of a woman was constructed between 2011 and 2013. 'Woman of Words' was created to celebrate the life and literary work of New Zealand's foremost woman writer, Katherine Mansfield. The artist describes her sculpture as a 'powerful warrior figure, wrapped in a close-fitting garment of quotations'. (retrieved from www.virginiakingsculptor.com/#/woman-of-words/). These quotations are from Katherine Mansfield's journals and short stories.

Like the sculpture, many women survivors of childhood sexual abuse wear the inscribed memories of the past as they go about their daily routines. They may not have the words to describe their experiences, or they may have learned to minimise what has happened in childhood and adolescence in order to continue their lives. Women survivors whose childhood trauma was unspeakable owing to the earliness of their abuse and/or the extent of their traumatisation can feel dissatisfied with aspects of their current life. This dissatisfaction may motivate them to see a helping professional to deal with the ongoing legacy of their abuse. Although the language or words might have been lacking initially, they may have retained some memories of their abuse. In the therapeutic relationship, these women may be supported to evolve the words to describe what has happened to them in the past. This ongoing dialogue with a professional helper may be important as life events continue to pose new challenges for women survivors, requiring reflection on their pasts for answers, resolution, and new directions to move forward.

Who this book is for

This preface introduces the anticipated audience and the aims and approaches that will be adopted throughout this book. The story of how the idea for the book developed is discussed, and the author's professional interest in the topic is clarified. The general pattern of each chapter is offered, with an opening quotation capturing the essence of what is to follow. Each chapter concludes by case examples to illustrate major points. The case studies presented are composites of many cases the author has encountered over her career, which spans over 30 years. The reader is reminded to pace his/her reading of each chapter to allow time for reflection and application in his/her own experience and clinical practice. The preface concludes with a chapter-by-chapter analysis of the structure of the book to prepare the reader for what is to follow.

This book is written to help professionals, including therapists and friends and families of women survivors of child sexual abuse (hereafter referred to using the abbreviation CSA), who wish to better understand the importance of disclosure in the recovery from historical sexual abuse. Within the chapters, I refer to readers as two different kinds of helpers: first, those who are informal providers of care to survivors of CSA, such as friends and family. Second, I refer to professional helpers, who include therapists, health practitioners, counsellors and clinical social workers, among others to whom women may choose to disclose.

In this preface, I will introduce myself as author and review some of the experiences that have been influential in the development of my interest in the theme of disclosure in my clinical work.

Readers are reminded of the potential for becoming vicariously traumatised by the content of the case studies; therefore, a paced approach to the reading is suggested to allow time for reflection on the practitioner's own experiences and case. If needed, seeking peer support, clinical supervision or one's own therapy is recommended for any issues that might be triggered by engagement with the material presented throughout the chapters.

How this book came to be

As I write this preface and embark on the writing of this book, the issue of disclosure of sexual abuse and harassment of women by men is prominent in media reports. At Oscar ceremonies in Hollywood, California, a public disclosure of abuse has ignited media interest in the ways in which power and secrecy can shroud the effects of a life impacted by sexual misconduct. One actress followed by another chose to disclose her own story of sexual abuse and harassment by the same director. Other women have since continued to come forward with similar claims, sharing their stories of harassment, intimidation and sexual abuse. What had remained an open secret in Hollywood has now been revealed as the underbelly of a professional community. Women came forward after Gwyneth Paltrow's now famous public disclosure which alleged the events involved a well-known and esteemed Hollywood director. The chain of events began with the retweeting of a hashtag, #MeToo, by actress Alyssa Milano who has encouraged other women in the entertainment industry to go public on the issue.

What has been remarkable about this series of events is that, through the solidarity of women disclosing in the public arena, these collective actions have suddenly exposed the sexist attitudes and misuse of power across the profession and within our society. Other men have been revealed as enablers or accomplices supporting either the survivor or the sexual misconduct of the alleged perpetrator. A community of support surrounding victims, both from women and men, within and without the acting profession, has enabled other adult women to have the courage to come forward to disclose on social media the abuse that happened in their lives. So the #MeToo process began and has grown into an international, online community of support for women who have been the victims of sexual abuse, harassment and misconduct.

Whether disclosure of sexual abuse is advisable or even necessary to healing from sexual and other forms of abuse is a question that has confounded the therapeutic literature over many years, beginning with the feminist and self-help movements of the 1970s and 1980s and the cautions of the New Trauma Therapy of the 1990s to mid-2000s, out of which developed modern-day understandings of trauma-informed therapy. What now seems clear is that women need to have a sense of their own power and autonomy to know that they have the choice to make the decision to disclose or not to disclose. This decision to disclose is affirmed and made in relationship to a caring significant or professional other. Many complex, systemic, cultural and contextual factors are at the heart of this decision as to whether to disclose or not. These factors are increasingly important in the work of therapists and other helping professionals who hear women disclose historical sexual abuse experienced during childhood that continues to impact their daily lives.

To disclose or not to disclose, or is that the right question?

These events reported in the media and the snowballing of allegations of the impact of abuse on adult women in the public consciousness raise the issue of what purpose disclosure has in the healing trajectory for women; what forms disclosure can take; and what enables or facilitates disclosure to occur safely for the survivor. Much of my professional life has involved listening to women disclose experiences of abuse and neglect. Chapter by chapter, I will provide an overview of the contexts in which I have worked, framing my abiding and long-standing interest in the topic of disclosure and its relationship to women's recovery from CSA.

As a mental health professional, during routine assessments with women referred by their general practitioners with symptoms of anxiety and depression, I saw many adult women in that context who referred to a past history of sexual assault during their childhood and/or adolescence. Often the past difficulties were re-experienced owing to life events in the present such as relationship difficulties, pregnancy, post-natal depression, work problems and interpersonal conflict within the extended family. Oftentimes, the perpetrator was reported to be a close family member. Poverty, health and housing difficulties often were secondary effects of CSA in adulthood, consistent with the research literature on the aftermath of CSA, which disrupts the life trajectory (Alaggia et al., 2019). Prompted by seeing the effects of CSA on adult women's mental health, I later began work in a national trauma unit where, for ten years, I read and listened to many hundreds of women's disclosures of abuse ranging from sexual grooming for molestation to sexual assault, incest and rape, in childhood and adolescence. I was mindful of how many adult women survivors of CSA moved into relationships that were abusive in adulthood. The ongoing legacy of CSA was highlighted across the lifespan in this clinical work. I came to realise that CSA led to further problems in adult relationships, impacting education, work, choice of partner and career. Within the rehabilitation unit that dealt with sexual abuse nationally in New Zealand, women disclosed experiences of sexual abuse in the past to their case managers and counsellors, and these disclosures formed the basis for a claim for mental injury known as a 'sensitive claim'. The accepted claim provided treatment services ranging from individual counselling to inpatient care. Without disclosure, it was not possible to determine eligibility for a sensitive claim, as the schedules of the Crimes Act necessitated assessment of the nature of the abuse described and a professional's opinion on the lasting impact of the abuse. In this sense, disclosure could open the door to opportunities for professional help in the community at a subsidised cost to the claimant.

After leaving that frontline of clinical practice, I changed to teaching and educating as an associate professor of social work for a further ten years, building on my experiences of working in the field. I had researched and completed a PhD while working in clinical practice. Being an academic enabled me to continue to research and write in this area, including publishing a book on the subject of vicarious traumatisation or the vicarious impact of the work on sexual abuse counsellors (Pack, 2016).

When I returned from academic life in Australia, I was keen to reconnect with the world of practice. This led to my taking a leadership role in a metropolitan hospital setting which involved assisting women to make complex decisions about pregnancy, and pregnancy loss. This lead counsellor position jettisoned me into grief and loss counselling across women's health. While leading a team of specialist counsellors and social workers, I was again faced with the harsh realities of women's lives, which often involved childhood abuse leading to ongoing experiences of abuse in adult relationships. Ambivalence about a current pregnancy often was about the woman's own early childhood or adolescent experiences. There was a wish to break the cycle of abuse, violence or poverty, and social isolation in the decision to seek counselling help. Again, I was aware of the wider implications of childhood sexual abuse in women's current lives. This was evident in the decision making of the woman survivor who was pregnant and presenting for assistance with decision making surrounding a pregnancy. I also began a new grief and loss counselling service for those women who experienced abnormality in pregnancy, ambivalence about news of a pregnancy, miscarriage, still birth, infertility and neonatal demise. I was reminded of how decision making around the right partner often meant delaying pregnancy. This delay introduced many complex psychosocial and genetic factors into the mix of presenting issues. While abuse was not always the primary reason for the delay, sometimes an ambivalence about, or decision to delay, pregnancy did have an underlying history of childhood sexual abuse or other forms of abuse.

These experiences, therefore, prompted my thinking about the need to begin to investigate how therapists and other helping professionals, across a range of helping professions, dealt with the issue of historical childhood sexual abuse and disclosure with adult women survivors of CSA. I was mindful that these historical issues may have arisen in a stage of life that posed new challenges, reigniting unresolved matters from the past. Whether or how we can assist survivors and their supporters to navigate the difficult and often complex decision making about whether to disclose childhood sexual abuse or not was raised in the research literature. The timing of when to disclose, how to safely disclose and, finally, to whom to disclose are some of the central questions raised from a therapeutic perspective.

To begin to address these questions, I first needed to research the meaning given to the process of disclosure in the therapeutic literature on sexual abuse recovery. With that understanding framing the discussion, the next issue was to determine how far disclosure can be seen as a necessary precursor to healing and rebounding from past abuse. I discovered in the past research that there is a gap in the literature on the role and place of disclosure in sexual abuse recovery by adult women survivors of CSA The existing research seemed to assume that disclosure was central to healing, as the mental health of women is considered to be compromised by the continuing legacy of CSA experiences if unaddressed (Schilling et al., 2007). In fact, the decision to disclose earlier abuse or not is a very complex and individual decision. It is not a singular event but a process that happens over time, often a lifetime (Alaggia, 2004; Alaggia, 2005). Women's choices and decision making around disclosure of historical CSA are considered to be influenced by age, life stage, culture and whether a trusting relationship is available in which sufficient emotional safety and scaffolding exist to support the process of disclosure (Brazelton, 2011; Brazelton, 2015; Brits et al., 2022). Conversely, difficulties with reporting to the authorities due to systems not communicating well across sectors or not operating easily for the survivor to navigate, cultural taboos against disclosure, and unfolding legal complexities in making a retrospective disclosure can derail, confound or significantly delay the process (Chenier et al., 2021). Therefore, attending to context in the decision whether to disclose experiences of CSA is now seen as being central to our understanding of the complexity of the process for survivors. What is missing in the research literature is an integrated approach to disclosure taking a comprehensive view of the relational, socio-cultural and life narrative factors involved in the decision making about disclosure of CSA.

Aims of the book

This book aims to bridge this gap in the existing literature on disclosure in women's healing from CSA. This understanding is necessary to evolve understandings of the impact of trauma and the role of disclosure in the healing trajectory. Towards this goal, this book will draw from both the insights from the research literature on sexual abuse recovery and these insights will be illustrated by case narratives. Themes from the research literature will draw from historical and classic texts and compare and contrast these with more recent research findings.

The intention of this book is to add to the limited knowledge base regarding the "disclosure process" among survivors of childhood sexual abuse and to identify what helps or hinders this process. The application of the life course and narrative approaches as a synthesis can be used to increase understanding of the factors influencing the process of disclosure. A life course perspective can provide a foundation for the development of age-related and culturally sensitive practice for women, children and families impacted by historical CSA.

The focus on women's experience is made owing to the prevalence of sexual abuse inflicted on women during childhood and adolescence across cultures and the life trajectory (Brazelton, 2011; Brazelton, 2015). This is not to suggest men and gender diverse communities do not have their own experiences of CSA to address, as the literature on male and gender diverse survivors continues to report themes that run in parallel to the issues for women. The lived experiences for women can be seen as distinct owing to women's socialisation and gender stereotypes which can prevent disclosure and, ultimately, healing from the effects during adulthood. Gilligan's founding work discusses how girls' and women's socialisation into a guiding 'ethic of care' predisposes women to placing the needs of others before their own, which can lead to an accommodation to and minimisation of abuse (Gilligan, 1982) . This is why the #MeToo movement is an important development as it established online communities of interest in which survivors of abuse felt supported to tell their stories of sexual abuse. Key theorists of women survivors' disclosure process have found the #MeToo movement to be a facilitating factor in changing societal attitudes about disclosure of CSA internationally (Alaggia & Wang, 2020).

Therefore, the aim of this book will be to define what childhood sexual abuse is, and how and why retrospective or historical disclosure of CSA is often made by women. What disclosure can involve will be further defined in terms of the types of disclosure or forms that disclosure can take. The term 'survivor' is used throughout this book rather than 'victim' to align with the current thinking about women's healing trajectory being re-authored from victim to survivor of CSA over the lifespan.

I will identify the individual, contextual and environmental factors that impede and facilitate disclosure of past abuse experiences, drawing from the evidence-based research literature on disclosure of CSA. The many forms that disclosure can take (from verbal to non-verbal) will be outlined and explained. The theoretical approaches to dealing with disclosure from adult women who have a history of CSA will be reviewed with reference to a literature review on women's experience of CSA in relation to disclosure. This review will provide the rationale for adopting a narrative, life course and relational perspective to the issue of disclosure and explore its role in the healing process.

A narrative, relational and life course perspective

A life course and narrative approach to disclosure across the stages of life will be adopted, where the usual transitions of each life stage trigger new challenges that need to be addressed and revisited over time in terms of the past childhood trauma. These same key life junctures often trigger new situations that bring adult women survivors to seek help from a significant other, therapist or counselling professional. How the therapist assesses the need to have conversations about disclosure will be introduced, and the various definitions of disclosure in the therapeutic relationship will be discussed. How therapists, from these conversations with adult women survivors, manage the disclosure process collaboratively with the survivor is critical to positive therapeutic outcomes for the woman survivor who may present at times of crisis or life transition. Narrative theory's focus on the major story having various subplots within it tells us much about why some storylines remain hidden and untold and others are partially told. Narrative theory assists us in identifying how such subplots fit with the major story. While there might have been disclosures of historical abuse and neglect prior to the current presentation to therapy, each life transition poses what I have conceptualised as a 'choice point' to disclose or to disclose again within a current life challenge. These 'choice points' propel survivors into an unknown zone, or what I discuss as being a 'liminal space' (Myerhoff, 1982; Myerhoff, 1992) in which deliberations are made by the survivor, on her own or with others, about the subplot of the CSA within the story of her life. The concept of liminal space within narrative theory was defined by the late cultural anthropologist Barbara

Myerhoff (Myerhoff, 1982; Myerhoff, 1992). 'Liminal spaces' are commonly encountered within one's life trajectory and are typically illuminated by key milestones and processes in which one looks at one's present life situation while reflecting on the past. Such milestones along the life trajectory often pose a need for a reiteration or a retelling of one's earlier history in the presence of another (Myerhoff, 1982; Myerhoff, 1992). Thus, earlier disclosures of CSA may require reflection and retelling so that another layer or depth of disclosure can be added as demanded by the challenge of a new situation(s) that is a feature of one's current life. The opportunity to explore, reflect and, in some cases, rework past trauma is presented again, bringing the potential for a new dimension of growth within the current life stage.

The structure of this book

Each chapter of this book aims to build upon the preceding one to develop a framework for working with disclosures of CSA by adult women survivors, within the context of the woman's biography and background. The issues of non-disclosure and delayed disclosure will be explored within each chapter as the context of disclosure is now thought to be more fluid and shifting than previously thought (Alaggia, 2004). The time being 'right' to disclose involves a coalescing of risk and protective factors in the face of a current challenge. In such a situation, there may be an opportunity to disclose or to disclose again, within a situation of relational safety, to a trusted adult. This opportunity can represent a 'choice point' for the woman survivor to decide to engage or not in the process of telling or retelling her story of CSA. This story is often about what happened in terms of the original CSA and the ongoing impact of the abuse on her life.

As with all research, the starting point is to define and review the relevance of concepts and theories in the research literature in relation to the decision making process in disclosure.

In Chapter One, the historical context in which theory developed to work with women survivors of sexual abuse will be overviewed. The research literature indicates that over half of adult women sexual abuse survivors delay disclosing for many years after the events, and a proportion will never disclose their abuse experiences to anyone, often owing to key socio-cultural factors (Alaggia, 2004; Brazelton, 2015). However, there is now an evidence base forming in the research literature about what conditions are needed for a woman survivor of CSA to feel safe enough to disclose to another. The relationship and the ability to form a safe attachment are paramount among these factors. A relationship of safe attachment is considered to be necessary to the disclosure of CSA (Brits et al., 2022). The historical framing of the New Trauma Therapy will be overviewed to explain how trauma-informed theory has developed with its relational focus.

Chapter Two will outline the importance of a narrative, life course perspective. This chapter aims to explain how historical abuse can impact at various stages of the life cycle. Variables, such as the woman's relationship with her early caregivers and peers, experiences of schooling, career, income and occupation, partnerships and relationships, will be explored as potential protective factors across the lifespan. Such resources will be analysed alongside the risk factors, which will be explored using previous research. The role of disclosure and its benefits and cautions will be reviewed with reference to the literature on sexual abuse recovery for adult women survivors of CSA.

In Chapter Three, with reference to the literature and models, the importance of prior attachments and relationships to establishing safety for the survivor to disclose will be explored. An expanded definition of disclosure is suggested. The conceptualisation of disclosure patterns, to include a range of relational, behavioural and indirect verbal and non-verbal attempts, will be summarised as 'different ways of telling' (McElvaney, 2015). Examples of intentionally withheld disclosures and disclosures that are triggered by flashbacks and memories of abuse, as well as dissociation as impacting disclosure of CSA, will be highlighted. One of the core therapeutic tasks is to facilitate opportunities for disclosure of CSA in order that the survivor client can construct a life narrative that explains and ultimately integrates these fragments into a coherent whole.

The chapter will conclude that an expanded conceptualisation of disclosure and the forms that disclosure can take across the lifespan provides professionals with a framework to understand and respond to adult survivors' disclosures more effectively.

Chapters Four, Five and Six will address different stages of the life cycle in terms of the developmental tasks evoking a need to disclose, or to revisit past disclosures of, CSA for women survivors. The cases used in these chapters are composite cases rather than relating to one actual case to avoid identifying a particular client. These case studies aim to illustrate the ways in which interpersonal, career and/or relationship difficulties, decisions about parenting or to remain single, pregnancy, birth and loss of pregnancy, parenting, health issues and growing older all impact in their potential to prompt grieving for the childhood that was not experienced. Mid years and later life will be explored with reference to the need to disclose CSA or to disclose it again to give new directions to these phases of life.

Chapter Seven focuses on the challenges of the global COVID-19 pandemic and the way the government restrictions imposed internationally have transformed our employing organisations, work routines and, hence, the way we work with women survivors of CSA. This may be a time women need to revisit past recollections of CSA owing to facing the challenges of being locked down with memories of past abuse as well as current challenges in a relationship. Helping professionals working with women survivors through remote and distant technologies necessitates new platforms on which the therapeutic relationship can be forged. The various challenges of using online technologies, often from home, are part of the new normal of the current world we live in, and so exploring the practicalities of doing this work from home and out of the office needs preparation, IT assistance and funding. The potential for vicarious traumatisation and difficulties with moving the clinical supervision of practice into a parallel online environment are explored with implications for future planning.

Chapter Eight explores the implications of the previous chapters for one's practice with women survivors of CSA. It concludes with a multi-theoretical and multidimensional model for working with disclosure from women survivors of CSA across the lifespan.

With this explanation setting the scene for what is to come, I will turn in the next chapter to defining core concepts and outlining the theoretical background justifying the life course approach to the topic.

I hope you will find this book a useful resource in your professional knowledge base. I wish you well with supporting your clients' decisions surrounding the disclosure of CSA in your clinical practice.

Dr Margaret Pack

References

Alaggia, R. (2004). Many ways of telling: expanding conceptualizations of child sexual abuse disclosure. *Child Abuse and Neglect*, 28, 1213–1227.

Alaggia, R. (2005). Disclosing the trauma of child sexual abuse: a gender analysis. *Journal of Trauma and Loss*, 10(5), 453–470.

Alaggia, R., Collin-Vezina, D., & Lateef, R. (2019). Facilitators and barriers to child sexual abuse (CSA) disclosures: a research update (2000–2016). *Trauma Violence Abuse*, 20(2), 260–283. doi:10.1177/1524838017697312

Alaggia, R., & Wang, S. (2020). 'I never told anyone until the #metoo movement': what can we learn from sexual abuse and sexual assault disclosures made through social media? *Child Abuse and Neglect*, 103. doi:10.1016/j.chiabu.2019.104312

Brazelton, J. (2011). African American women looking back: making meaning of the disclosure process of incest survivors across the life course. *Dissertation Abstracts International: Section A. Humanities and Social Sciences*, 72(2-A), 738.

Brazelton, J. F. (2015). The secret storm: exploring the disclosure process of African American women survivors of child sexual abuse across the life course. *Traumatology*, 21(3), 181.

Brits, B., Walker-Williams, H., & Fouche, A. (2022). Experiences of women survivors of childhood sexual abuse in relation to nonsupportive significant adults: a scoping review. *Trauma Violence Abuse*, 23(4), 1027–1047. doi:10.1177/1524838020985550

Chenier, K., Shawyer, A., Williams, A., & Milne, R. (2021). 'Cold feet': the attrition of historic child sexual abuse cases reported to the police in a Northern Canadian Territory. *Child Abuse and Neglect*, 120. doi:10.1016/j.chiabu.2021.105206

Gilligan, C. (1982). *In A Different Voice: Psychological Theory and Women's Development*. Harvard University Press.

McElvaney, R. (2015). Disclosure of child sexual abuse: delays, non-disclosure and partial disclosure. What the research tells us and implications for practice. *Child Abuse Review*, 24(3), 159–169. doi:10.1002/car.2280

Myerhoff, B. G. (1982). *Number Our Days: Triumph of Continuity and Culture among Jewish Old People in an Urban Ghetto*. Simon & Schuster/Touchstone Books.

Myerhoff, B. G. (1992). *Remembered Lives: The Work of Ritual, Story Telling and Growing Older*. University of Michigan Press.

Pack, M. (2016). *Self-Help for Trauma Therapists: A Practitioner's Guide*. Routledge.

Schilling, E. A., Aseltine, R. H., Jr., & Gore, S. (2007). Adverse childhood experiences and mental health in young adults: a longitudinal survey. *BMC Public Health*, 7. doi:10.1186/1471-2458-7-30

1 Theoretical approaches underpinning disclosure of CSA by women

Introduction

In this chapter, the historical context in which theory was developed to work with adult survivors of childhood sexual abuse will be overviewed, together with the prevalence of CSA. The role of disclosure will then be explored within these theoretical frameworks. A working definition of sexual abuse is offered, acknowledging that there are many forms of abuse. Physical, emotional, psychological and sexual abuse, along with neglect in childhood, are now understood to often occur concurrently and, therefore, are seen as being inseparable from each other. As they often occur together, they are considered as being interlocking in their effects and impact on the survivor. With this understanding, each kind of abuse forms a part of the childhood traumatic experience as a whole.

As there are few clear definitions of many of the terms used when describing disclosure, recollecting the abuse retrospectively and the recovery process, an attempt is made to clarify some working definitions from the research literature. From current thinking about sexual abuse recovery, the historical roots of trauma-informed theory are explored in relation to the New Trauma Therapy.

The chapter concludes with a case study from my practice in the mid-1980s when there was little integrated trauma theory about the role of disclosure in women's healing from CSA. As this was the first time I had encountered a woman client who wished to disclose CSA to me, this disclosure was representative as being a 'first telling' (Gasker, 1999). Gasker (1999) writes of the power of initial disclosures of CSA in terms of its impact both for the woman who discloses and for the worker who hears the disclosure. Rather than being a glowing example of my practice, the case study of Fiona speaks of the difficulty of knowing how to deal with and manage one's own traumatic transference and vicarious traumatisation while endeavouring to stay connected and to engage with the woman's disclosure. Furthermore, the case study speaks to having a clinical supervisor who was unaware of the complexity of the psychodynamic processes underlying disclosure of CSA as these themes had yet to be expounded in a coherent trauma-informed theory at this time.

DOI: 10.4324/9781032669205-1

To frame this case study, I will begin with a description of how I approached the literature review on women's disclosure of CSA.

Search strategy

To research the issue of CSA disclosure in sexual abuse recovery for adult women, I searched for relevant literature using the keywords women OR female, disclosure AND attachment AND 'sexual abuse' in PsycInfo for 2005–2018 and Social Services Abstracts 2010–2018. As well as using this date range as a delimiter, the search was limited in terms of whether the articles were available in the English language. Most articles were found in the multidisciplinary, multicultural/international context and were peer reviewed for rigour. A variety of research papers were found, including randomised controlled trials, small case studies and evaluations, and larger quantitative studies of entire geographic populations. Once the search was run and hits were found in the searched electronic databases, the abstracts were read for relevance, and the themes were analysed. These themes were then synthesised for reporting. This search was supplemented by the classic works establishing the trauma-informed theory we know and use today. This was the first main search informing the research for this book and took place in the years of researching and writing the book, which spanned the years 2018–2024.

To set the wider context for the book, I begin in the next section with a working definition of child sexual abuse. With that understanding established, I will summarise what is known about the factors that impact adult women's disclosure, drawn from the recent research literature.

What is child sexual abuse?

Child sexual abuse is defined in various ways in the research and practice literature; however, recent definitions commonly identify the power imbalance between the survivor and abuser, as illustrated in the World Health Organization's guidelines on child sexual abuse:

> Child sexual abuse is the involvement of a child in sexual activity that he or she does not fully comprehend, is unable to give informed consent to, or for which the child is not developmentally prepared and cannot give consent, or that violates the laws or social taboos of society. Child sexual abuse is evidenced by this activity between a child and an adult or another child who by age or development is in a relationship of responsibility, trust or power, the activity being intended to gratify or satisfy the needs of the other person. This may include but is not limited to: – the inducement or coercion of a child to engage in any unlawful sexual activity; – the exploitative use of a child in prostitution or other unlawful sexual practices; – the exploitative use of children in pornographic performance and materials.
>
> (WHO, 2017, 7.1)

In my clinical experience, a child's witnessing of adult sexual acts falls within the scope of child sexual abuse when there may be no direct physical touching or even intentional involvement under the Crimes Act 1961 (Ministry of Justice, New Zealand, 1961), the Act we would refer to when considering claims for compensation and treatment expenses through the Accident Compensation and Rehabilitation Corporation (ACC). The ACC is a publicly funded, no-faults rehabilitation scheme in New Zealand the aim of which is to compensate injured persons, including the victims of childhood sexual abuse and adult sexual assault. Assessing the initial sensitive claim for ACC eligibility determined whether the sexual abuse fitted the descriptions of the schedules of sexual abuse under the Crimes Act 1961. Under the provisions of a 'sensitive claim' for mental injury, there needed to be evidence from a counsellor or other health professional that the abuse as described had occurred and had an aftermath for the claimant if it had occurred in the past. Non-contact sexual abuse – for example, when an adolescent girl is observed showering by an older male relative or house guest in her home for his sexual gratification – would be regarded under New Zealand law as an incident of child sexual abuse owing to the mental injury inflicted on the victim by a responsible adult's actions. The power imbalance due to the age of the perpetrator and his relationship to the adolescent also fits the World Health Organization (WHO) definition of CSA. Therefore, it is not essential for there to be any physical contact, as this example illustrates. In the case of children exposed to pornographic material online, owing to the differing maturity and power imbalance between child and adult, this would also be considered as sexual abuse under New Zealand law and, therefore, can be compensated under a sensitive claim for mental injury.

To summarise, in the context of this book, CSA is defined as any act involving a child that is intended to provide sexual gratification to a parent, caregiver or other older individual who has responsibility for the child. Childhood sexual abuse, drawing on the American Psychiatric Association definition, includes a range of activities such as fondling a child's genitals, penetration, incest, rape, sodomy and indecent exposure (APA, 2013). There is a higher reported prevalence among girls who disclose historical abuse as women (Lahav & Elklit, 2016). This trend was affirmed when New Zealand's *Next Magazine* commissioned a national survey into the issue and found that 28% of all women surveyed in New Zealand had been sexually assaulted at some point in their lives. Whether to disclose what happened to a trusted significant other continued to be an issue for those women *Next Magazine* surveyed, with the #MeToo movement giving some of the women surveyed the solidarity to speak up about what happened in the past (Bennett, 2018). But what is disclosure for women survivors, and why is it important in the healing from CSA?

Disclosure and the timing of disclosure

When a person tells another some highly private and personal information, perhaps material that threatens the reputation of powerful adult(s), it is as though they are telling a long-kept secret, one that should not be told, often because of threats made by the perpetrator or an anticipated negative response from the person to whom disclosure is made. In the telling, survivors of CSA are considered to have disclosed something about themselves, their life and their relationship with the perpetrator. Whether or not the listener to the disclosure affirms and remains supportive of what is said is the variable often discussed in recent literature on the role and impact of disclosure of CSA. How disclosure or lack of disclosure plays out in the healing from past trauma is central to our understanding in the field of sexual abuse recovery for women survivors. Therefore, the notion of there being a safe attachment to the person who is being disclosed to – that is, one who is deemed to be trustworthy by the survivor – is considered to be the paramount consideration. This assessment of trustworthiness to be a confident is a theme regardless of whether this person is a professional helper, friend or family member (McElvaney, 2015).

The point is made by the World Health Organization (WHO) in the 2017 guidelines on sexual abuse of children that, unlike the disclosure of sexual abuse by adult women, children generally do not disclose at the time of the abuse. There are several reasons for this decision to delay disclosure or not to disclose. First, disclosure tends to be a process rather than a single event and is often prompted following a physical health issue or behavioural concern in which a health professional becomes aware of a condition that requires treatment. The second main reason for delayed disclosure or non-disclosure is related to the fact that the perpetrator may have threatened to harm the child who then goes through life with the knowledge that, if they disclose, there will be recriminations or threats of harm to themself or others. WHO acknowledges the complexity of assessing children for child sexual abuse and specifies that working with child clients requires special skills and techniques in assessment which might need to involve forensic interviewing, police investigation and physical/psychological examination. The practitioner facing these roles may also need to address specific issues related to consent to enable information to be shared among other health practitioners and authorities for the welfare of the child. The role may span the reporting of child sexual abuse, so that others who are not formally trained may be required to undertake specialist assessment (WHO, 2017).

The implications for the disclosure of sexual abuse in childhood or adolescence retrospectively, therefore, is fraught with difficulty. The complexity of what constitutes a disclosure varies, as it is difficult to define. Coercion and threats to keep a secret are often involved. Therefore, a description of the context surrounding the events, which may have occurred many years ago with trusted parental caregivers, is needed. Accuracy of remembering what happened can be an issue when disclosing owing to the fragmented nature of traumatic memory. Telling for the first time may differ from subsequent telling, and, thus, disclosure is thought to grow over time in the remembering of traumatic memory. For these reasons, disclosure of CSA by adult women is now conceptualised as being a discursive and iterative process that occurs across time. It can be circular rather than linear in nature, as talking about one's abuse may trigger further memories from the past in an attempt at making sense of what happened. In this way, disclosure may grow in the telling (Alaggia, 2004).

The research literature indicates that over half adult women sexual abuse survivors delay disclosing for many years after the events, and, furthermore, a proportion of women survivors will never disclose their abuse experiences to anyone (Brazelton, 2015; McElvaney, 2015). However, there is now an evidence base in the research literature of some of the factors that may prevent disclosure, as well as those that may assist it. This literature optimistically predicts disclosure as a first step towards healing for CSA survivors. The factors that are thought of as facilitators of or obstacles to the disclosure of CSA will be outlined next with reference to the related concepts of 'recovery', 'dissociation' and 'resilience'.

The pervasive nature of sexual abuse for women

In the North American context, 30% of adult women seeking health treatment have been found to have a history of some form of abuse in childhood (Becker et al., 2010). In particular, psychological and sexual abuse have been shown to predict PTSD symptoms across the research literature. The interlocking nature of different forms of abuse – physical, psychological and sexual – are also demonstrated across the studies (Becker et al., 2010). Authors have argued that looking separately at each form of abuse (physical, sexual and psychological abuse and neglect) may contribute to health care professionals' understanding of the mental health consequences and sequelae of sexual abuse (Bottoms et al., 2014). Some studies demonstrate a higher risk of intimate partner violence (IPV) for women reporting psychological abuse (Giacci et al., 2022). Other studies demonstrate the longer-term impact of childhood sexual abuse compared to physical abuse as discrete experiences that have distinct, identifiable impacts (Glover et al., 2010). Yet other studies have found that each form of childhood abuse foreshadows similar consequences in adulthood. Regardless of the nature of the abuse, there are identifiable impacts, with severe repeated CSA being associated with longer-term consequences in adulthood (Gupta et al., 2011).

IPV is considered to be one of the frequently encountered adult consequences of having a history of childhood sexual abuse, across many cultures (Jeremiah et al., 2017). The intergenerational consequences for mothers and daughters who have been sexually abused earlier in life and then have gone on to choose partners who replicate patterns of abuse towards them in adulthood have been highlighted in some studies, cross-culturally and over several generations (Giacci et al., 2022; Glover et al., 2010; Jeremiah et al., 2017; Rueda et al., 2021; Simmel et al., 2012).

Although there is a view that experiencing adult IPV where childhood abuse is present can compound the symptoms of complex PTSD experienced, there is increasing evidence from a life course perspective that looks at experiences of abuse across the lifespan. This broader view may better guide professionals from whom women survivors of CSA seek care. Research suggests that women who experience CSA are two to ten times more likely to experience IPV as adults when compared to those adult women not abused in childhood (Becker et al., 2010, p. 1701). However, various protective factors, the presence of which are considered to act as buffers for the more negative life events, are now thought to lead to variations in the impact of CSA in adulthood. We will explore the balance of risk and protective factors related to having a history of CSA in this and forthcoming chapters. Differing theoretical perspectives from which a practitioner works may also mean that they distinguish the legacy of CSA in adult women differently. Guided by different mixes of theoretical approaches to working with women CSA survivors – which theories a helping clinician selects and works from – impacts how CSA and its aftermath are viewed. The rest of this chapter will explore this reference to differing theoretical approaches in work with women survivors of CSA.

The impact of CSA and its legacy in adulthood

It is difficult to distinguish the impact of early child sexual abuse on one's life in adulthood in part owing to the many ways of approaching the understanding of sexual abuse and the aftermath of such a history. In my research with sexual abuse counsellors in the New Zealand context, I found that, to work in the area of sexual abuse recovery, it is necessary to draw on an eclectic mix of theories to inform one's practice (Pack, 2016). To begin with, historically, a feminist self-help orientation framed the early theorising of what helped recovery from CSA. Later understandings incorporated a staged approach known as the New Trauma Therapy, where disclosure and exploring memory were recommended once therapeutic safety was established and skills for moderating strong emotions were strengthened. Currently, trauma-informed theorising assesses the context of the woman's life and the balancing of risk and protective factors that inform the decision making about whether to disclose and engage in healing work.

Given the enormity of the transgression of personal boundaries that has occurred during a woman's experience of childhood sexual abuse, the central dilemma for the helping professional is: 'how can I meet the client's need for relationship and connection safely without triggering a reliving of what has happened in the distant past?' Second, if the occurrence of sexual abuse suggests unequal relationships in which power is misused and the survivor is denied her own subjectivity, how do we assist in the retrieval of the client's own voice? For many therapists and other helping professionals such as counsellors, psychotherapists and social workers, training is grounded in psychodynamic principles and practices that are originally based on psychoanalytic theory. Coupled with this, disclosure in the therapeutic context has been associated with attachment theory and, in particular, how to provide a holding or 'liminal space' (the space between the known and journeying into the unknown), in which the client can safely explore her personal narrative to integrate current life themes with what has happened earlier in her life. The influence of the New Trauma Theory, which is now no longer new, has been a paradigm shift, beginning in the 1990s, that has integrated several strands of theory, including feminist, social justice, and systemic theories of practice, to achieve an understanding. The New Trauma theorists recommended a paced and tailored approach to the circumstances of each woman who presents with historical CSA. These theorists posit that it is necessary to work collaboratively with each woman who presents for help with sexual abuse in the past to know where to start to assist the survivor. New Trauma Therapy provided the springboard for trauma-informed theory as we know it today, incorporating insights from neural brain development in children and neuroscience. Alongside these theoretical developments, the concept of 'recovery' exists. To understand the process of recovery, the allied terms of dissociation and resilience will be defined to show how understandings of these concepts have grown over time.

Recovery

The process of accessing and processing recollections of abuse and integrating what has happened in one's life narrative to understand one's life in the present is generally referred to as 'sexual abuse recovery'. Herman (1992), in her seminal work *Trauma and Recovery*, sets out one of the first comprehensive stages of healing from childhood sexual abuse for adult survivors. Reworking the classical work of the physician Pierre Janet, who worked intensively with women inpatients in French psychiatric asylums in the nineteenth century, Herman theorises a new way of working with women survivors of CSA. In a similar way to Freud, Janet worked with women who had been diagnosed with a condition known as 'hysteria' while, during their treatment in psychiatric asylums, they disclosed histories of being sexually abused during childhood. Janet advocated the practice of clinicians engaging women in 'talking therapy' for such presentations when containment was the main intervention with such diagnoses (Herman, 1992). Herman reports that Janet continued to work with women patients who had disclosed CSA by engaging them in hypnotic or trance sates. This was in contrast to Freud, who abandoned hypnosis at the time in favour of the therapist representing the 'blank screen' of psychoanalysis. Free association with the patient was to be encouraged in classical Freudian psychoanalysis (Freud, 1909). In historical accounts of Janet's work with women survivors of CSA, Herman (1992) finds an early theory of dissociation on which she builds her own theory for guiding practitioners who deal with women who have histories of CSA.

Dissociation

Dissociation is a term conceptualised by Herman and other proponents of the New Trauma Therapy, including Briere, Courtois and Dalenberg, in the 1990s and beyond. The New Trauma Therapists theorise that dissociation is a normal response to traumatic events in which the body continues to work as it does usually as though on automatic pilot, while inwardly the body is felt to be acting on its own, separated from the self in a dreamlike reality. Herman draws on the phenomenon of 'shell shock' experienced by soldiers returning from World War One to explain the concept of dissociation. Veterans described out-of-body experiences as a means of coping on a daily basis with life-threatening situations from which there was no relief or escape. The method of coping by a psychic withdrawal out of the body to exist in various states of altered consciousness informs Herman's theorising about women's survivors of CSA dissociating while recollecting their abuse. Theorists of the New Trauma Therapy, who include Herman (1992), Briere (1989), Courtois (1988) and Dalenberg (2000), all relate a knowledge and recognition of dissociative processes as being fundamental to our understanding of trauma and how to assist women survivors in a staged model of recovery. This is in contrast to some narrative therapists who find the use of the term 'dissociation' pathologising, and so they prefer alternative terminology to be used. Chapter Two will explore alternative understandings of dissociation from a narrative and life course perspective.

Two of the foundational comprehensive models for professionals working with the retrospective disclosures of women abused as children, along with Dr Judith Herman, were frameworks developed by Dr Christine Courtois (1997) and Dr John Briere (1989). As Courtois reports in reflecting on her early theorising on sexual abuse recovery, her orientation contrasted with the predominant perspectives of that time that minimised the impact of abuse and accounted for it by Freudian notions of disclosure as being associated with women's fantasies or wish fulfilment. Van der Kolk (van der Kolk et al., 1996) broadened and refined treatment models for working across differing traumatised populations to guide clinicians who had in their caseloads clients who had a range of traumatic experiences and responses.

In a similar way to Freudian theories, they conceptualised the recovery process as being very individual, gradual and not time-limited. But, unlike Freudian analytical thinking, recovery depended on building skills and strengthening personal resources before dealing with the processing of memories of the trauma. The stages of recovery conceptualised by Herman (1992) place an emphasis on establishing safety. Assessing the client's existing strengths is important in approaching what safety looks like for the client. This a problematic stage of treatment as, until safety is firmly established, the client is at risk of being re-traumatised by the past, as it can be re-experienced contemporaneously with the present, prompting regression back to childhood. If the client cannot sustain the emotional challenge of connecting with a helping professional, they may remain ambivalent about trusting again. If untrusting, the client may not engage or, alternatively, they may delay or drop out of contact.

Once safety has clearly been established from the woman's perspective, then disclosure through remembering, followed by a stage of mourning for the loss of innocence and childhood, is recommended. After the past is grieved for, which may arise at many points in a woman's life, triggered by usual milestone events, there may be a settling of the issues. This process of mourning, supported by helping professionals, may involve coming to a philosophic acceptance of an early life that was blighted by experiences of sexual abuse, tempered by looking forward to the present life in a world that has been forever changed. Ultimately, Herman (1992) advocates that the therapist begin to explore with the woman 're-connection with everyday life' (p. 155).

The factors that are assessed in terms of the personal resources of the woman survivor have been recently linked to protective factors that buffer the more negative impact of early childhood experiences. Most of the research on resilience has been developed from longitudinal studies of children who have thrived despite having experienced abuse and neglect. Resilience is a controversial concept when applied to women CSA survivors in terms of healing past trauma; however, there are strong connections with a quality of relationship that enables disclosure that is of current interest in the research literature.

Resilience

While much has been written about the short- and longer-term effects of sexual abuse, relatively little has been written about women survivor's resilience in comparison with the inevitable negative impacts of CSA. Across the studies reviewed by Domhardt, Münzer, Fegert and Goldbeck (2015), resilience is understood to be a dynamic concept involving the survivor's personal resources and personal characteristics as well as aspects of the survivor's social and familial context and life circumstances. Some studies have discovered the attainment of positive adaptation within the context of adversity from CSA, especially if there is some caregiver support from the non-offending parent or guardian (Wallis & Woodworth, 2021). Some theorists believe that adaptation in one area of life or domain is needed to indicate resilience; others conclude that positive adaptation to adversity across several domains of life is needed before resilience can be evidenced.

Thirty-seven articles relating to survivors of CSA were reviewed by Domhardt et al. (2015) who discovered that between 10% and 53% of survivors reported a level of functioning despite a history of sexual abuse. The existence of protective factors that buoyed survivors through adverse impacts from histories of CSA has been noted across the lifespan, from adolescence to later years. The protective factors identified include successful education and school experiences from primary to higher education; interpersonal and emotional intelligence; thinking that the locus of control rests with the survivor rather than others; active coping strategies including involvement in groups, interests and community; optimism about oneself and one's future life; and positive social attachment. Being able to shift self-blame and attribute blame to the perpetrator of the abuse is also considered a protective factor. In summary, the single most important protective factor discovered by the authors was the social support available from family, groups and community (Domhardt et al., 2015).

Facilitating support and encouraging survivors to take advantage of support that is offered suggest that both an individual/couple/family approach and, in some cases, a community approach to recovery from CSA are needed. This broader vision, together with a consciousness-raising, activist approach from practitioners to tackle negative stereotypes about abuse and the prevalence of CSA in society, is further recommended. Historically, paying attention to these systemic factors has been of central importance to therapists in their efforts to assist women survivors of CSA. A parallel development has been evident with the bringing into public consciousness the needs of returning war veterans who required assistance with rebuilding their lives after combat duty. The origins of the New Trauma Therapy of the mid-to-late 1980s recognised such parallels in developing a dual focus on both the individual and the society in which they live that itself needed to recognise and take responsibility for the aftermath of past traumatic experience at community and societal levels.

Setting the historical context: the role of disclosure, from Freud to the New Trauma Therapy

The war veterans returning from the two world wars made it more acceptable to disclose psychological impacts from trauma, though there were still difficulties with the authorities acknowledging the longer-term effects on the veterans' lives upon their re-entry into civilian and family life (Herman, 1992).

In an effort to compensate and rehabilitate the emerging traumatised and marginalised groups in society, such as war veterans and women, new ways of conceptualising the therapeutic relationship emerged in the 1970s. Out of the self-help and feminist movements of the 1960s and 1970s, acknowledgement of how women's socialisation and discrimination had shaped their experiences began to be openly discussed. The guide for women survivors of CSA, *The Courage to Heal*, first published in 1988 and revised and updated ever since, broke new ground as it asked women if they had been sexually abused; if so, the authors discussed options for healing (Bass & Davis, 1988; Bass & Davis, 1992). Such publications have fallen into disrepute since the False Memory Syndrome Foundation and affiliated bodies have accused therapists of implanting memories of abuse through reference to such resources (Courtois, 1997). Nonetheless, Bass and Davis established one of the most widely read self-help guides for women survivors of CSA following the earlier feminist guide: *Our Bodies, Ourselves* (Boston Women's Health Book Collective, 1976).

When practitioners were challenged by a need to respond to an increasing demand for appropriate guides for working with women survivors of CSA, they turned their attention to the existing theories of practice. Conceptual use was made of part of the original psychodynamic framework, particularly surrounding the transference–countertransference dyad and the therapeutic alliance; however, other Freudian ideas were challenged. In classical Freudian psychoanalysis, the therapeutic relationship between client and helping professional is predicated on the idea of the therapist representing the 'blank screen' on to which the patient projects all thoughts and emotions. The woman survivor is cast in the position of revealing the self, as both conscious and unconscious psychological material is evoked by the process that is contained within the relationship. The therapist, in contrast, is required to avoid all self-disclosure and remains emotionally distanced from the content of the material disclosed to maintain therapeutic neutrality. The psychoanalytic psychotherapist, like a medical physician, is the assessor and the initiator of diagnosis and treatment on the basis of expert knowledge.

Freud was never comfortable with his discovery that the origins of the diagnosis of 'hysteria', the archetypal female neurosis of his time, were located in a history of childhood sexual abuse. Early work by Freud on treating hysterical conversion symptoms through hypnosis led to the first hypotheses on psychodynamics and the search for methods other than hypnosis for bringing into consciousness repressed intrapsychic material. Initially, Freud concluded that hysteria was the result of traumatic sexual experiences associated with a large amount of emotion that was not able to be dissipated by the conscious mind but instead remained shored up in the unconscious mind, returning in the guise of various symptoms (see, for example, Freud, 1909). Memories of events such as incest were thought to be unacceptable to the conscious mind and so were repressed and in need of expression through hypnosis. Freud was later to disbelieve his women patients' disclosure of incest, locating the site of these disclosures as residing in the psychopathology of the individual (Dalenberg, 2000; Courtois, 1997).

Freud's repudiation of his own theories was a historical product of the times in which he lived. If Freud had admitted that incest and sexual abuse were as widely reported as he heard from his patients, he would have implied impropriety to a large proportion of respectable and powerful men in society. Perhaps realising the implications of his work with its implicit challenges to patriarchal values, he refused to identify men as sexual abusers, and within a year he repudiated his seduction theory entirely. His reframing of seduction theory involved his conclusion that women patients' reports of sexual abuse were untrue. As a kind of wish fulfilment, women survivors of CSA were seen as disclosing their abuse as fantasies based in their own incestuous desires.

In discovering the prevalence of the abuse of women during childhood, Freud promoted a belief in society about the untrustworthiness of women survivors' accounts of abuse. This belief continues to be deeply ingrained in society and in the culture of psychotherapy today. In an effort to challenge this culture of disbelief, feminist writers maintain a dual focus on the socialisation of women and girls as informing their moral reasoning. For example, Gilligan found girls' ethical decision making influenced by their ongoing assessment of the needs of others (Gilligan, 1982).

The bridge between Freudian and feminist responses to women's disclosures of CSA

Carol Gilligan was one of the psychologist researchers who provided a bridge between feminist critiques of Freudian psychoanalytic theory and the development of a feminist psychology that views women's psychology as being essentially different to men's as it is more relational, influenced by girls' socialisation to attend to and care for others before themselves (Gilligan, 1982). Like in Gilligan (1982) and Bass and Davis (1992), disclosure and healing from CSA for women survivors had a political as well as therapeutic meaning. The New Trauma Therapy that evolved represents a hybrid of psychodynamic concepts deriving from humanistic concerns that emphasised the need for the therapist, when working with women survivors, to 'bear witness' to CSA trauma on a societal as well as individual level and to engage in advocacy to change the status of women in society (Herman, 1992). For Herman, therapy was reconceptualised as having a social and political import, and, thus, the site of the therapeutic relationship itself is an act of political resistance and activism, challenging patriarchal systems and those who uphold systems that discriminate negatively against women. The experience of trauma is often beyond expression in words, and so the task of therapy is to grapple with alternative modes of expression of experiences that often are beyond the realms of normally lived experience for the therapist.

Another theorist in the tradition of the New Trauma Therapy, Dr Constance Dalenberg (2000), uses metaphor and poetry as alternative modes of articulating her clients' experiences in terms of disclosure of CSA. The challenge for the therapist is to find ways of enabling the survivor to articulate the unspeakable (Dalenberg, 2000).

Reformulating the therapeutic alliance

In a parallel way to feminist reconceptualisations of women's psychology, humanist traditions epitomised in the founding work of Carl Rogers (1995) and humanist contemporaries hypothesised that it was the experiential knowledge and personal growth of the therapist that were associated with what was considered to be necessary for the formation of the therapeutic relationship. The self of the therapist and all responses felt towards the client were thought to inform and shape the therapeutic alliance dynamically. For client-centred humanists such as Rogers, and the Gestalt tradition that viewed the qualities of genuineness and authenticity as the cornerstone of the therapeutic alliance, the therapeutic relationship itself provided the context for healing (Kahn, 1991). In such reconceptualisations, the self of the therapist became the main means of therapeutic transformation. It was the site in which the conditions conducive to the development of emotional safety through mutual trust and respect/power-sharing between client and therapist facilitate the disclosure of CSA and witness it on a broader societal stage. The Gestalt psychotherapists, beginning with Fritz Perls and his involvement in developing the encounter group movement during the 1960s and 1970s, set the stage for new ways of conceptualising knowledge that were in contrast to the therapist-as-scientist model. Humanist traditions of psychotherapy opened the door, metaphorically speaking, for a rapprochement of psychoanalytic thinking and alternative models of therapy that gave voice to the marginalised in western society. Within the humanistic tradition of the 1960s and 1970s, the experiences of women, combat veterans and ethnic/cultural minorities were accorded the same respect as other groups.

Kahn saw the 1960s and 1970s as throwing up numerous dilemmas for therapists who were pushed to make impossible choices at this time:

> So, theoretically there were two possible ways of being truly therapeutic: One could be considerably more engaged with one's patients than the rules permitted, or one could be an unusually warm and compassionate person with an unusual capacity to communicate that compassion. Actually, I believe, the analysts were caught in an impossible contradiction. On the one hand they required of themselves that they maintain a relatively severe neutrality, and on the other hand, they needed to create a therapeutic ambiance of trust, security and confidence.
>
> (Kahn, 1991, p. 8)

As with Rogers, Kahn and proponents of the New Trauma Therapy see the building of rapport with traumatised clients as a painstaking and crucial phase for client and therapist. As women survivors of CSA have personal experiences of deep betrayal, the task of rebuilding trust in another is fraught with potential pitfalls. Here, the notion of transference or the feelings and thoughts of the client about the therapist are central. For example, Herman's (1992) idea of transference taking on a 'life and death' quality conceptualised the ways in which the therapeutic relationship became the site for the re-experiencing of some of the woman's original experiences of trauma. Other theorists in the tradition of the New Trauma Therapy remark that the work with women survivors of CSA is no longer attributable to the client's innate characteristics or personality, but is more frequently related to the client's and therapist's respective responses to the traumatic themes and narratives that are evoked in therapy (Dalenberg, 2000). The therapeutic relationship, therefore, includes the sense or presence of the perpetrator. Therefore, the perpetrator is seen as a third participant in the therapeutic relationship (Dalenberg, 2000). In this way, 'traumatic transference', following Herman's (1992) conceptualisation of the term, represents more than the client–therapist dyad.

The relationship lives in the shadow of the perpetrator. As part of the client's process, it is inevitable that the projection of transference of the client's responses and feelings towards her perpetrator is at some point projected on to the therapist through the process of engagement in the therapeutic relationship. For therapists or other helping professionals who find themselves cast in the role of perpetrator, this can be a deeply challenging experience, but, as Herman (1992) astutely points out, such responses are to be expected and planned for.

To illustrate some of the themes of the therapeutic relationship and the nature of traumatic transference when dealing with adult women survivors of CSA, the following case example from my own practice is offered. As discussed in the preface, this case represents not a shining example of my practice but a historical example that preceded the introduction of comprehensive frameworks of trauma-informed theory such as the New Trauma Therapy. Rather, we were guided to use Bass and Davis's *The Courage to Heal* as a self-help guide with clients (Bass & Davis, 1988). Therefore, this description illustrates the patchy state of the existing knowledge base for practitioners working with women with CSA.

Case example: Fiona and 'old blue eyes'

Early in my career as a mental health social worker, in the late 1980s, there was a burgeoning awareness of the impact of CSA on women who presented at our community health clinic. One such referral was from a local general practitioner who mentioned that his patient had had persistent depressive or anxiety symptoms that had recurred at key moments; hence, the referral for advice for future management was sought from our multidisciplinary team of psychologists, psychiatrists, nurses, social workers and occupational therapists. The theoretical context of sexual abuse counselling in the 1980s was the feminist and self-help movements which suggested that disclosure and catharsis were the means of healing from traumatic events in the past. Our clinic adopted a standard question in the initial client assessment: 'Have you experienced abuse in your past?' By making explicit the unspeakable, many clients disclosed, at an early point in their contact, extensive histories of sexual, physical and psychological abuse. Using the structure of the self-help guide *The Courage to Heal* (Bass & Davis, 1988), I was aware of the distress that was evoked by remembering past traumatic material. Yet facilitating disclosure of past traumatic events was much recommended by theory at that time so that fragments of memory could be processed and finally integrated. Using Bass and Davis' approach, healing would be possible for the client, and they would be freed from reliving the past constantly with disclosure being encouraged. I am now mindful of the cautionary focus of the New Trauma Therapy suggesting skill building prior to any traumatic memory work.

One of the clients I worked with at the time I will refer to as Fiona. Fiona was a 27-year-old woman who had been referred to our clinic with symptoms of anxiety that prevented her keeping her employment. At the initial assessment, she disclosed a long history of incest at the hands of a step-parent who moved in to live with her mother in a lesbian partnership after her marriage to her husband had ended. Fiona had been groomed over her early teens by her stepmother who had moved from fondling to penetrating her vagina with objects. Fiona appeared distrustful at initial interview and described insomnia over many years. Later, I was to learn that her stepmother used to come into her bedroom at night to abuse her, hence her hypervigilance at night. She referred to her stepmother as 'old blue eyes', sometimes affectionately and at other times in a derogatory fashion. Fiona's ambivalent relationship with a parental figure who was sometimes loving and at others abusive, I hypothesised, would make my relationship with her ambivalent and unpredictable owing to the nature of her relationship with her stepmother and mother. Her mother was blamed for not knowing what was happening and for moving her stepmother into her home. Fiona had tried to disclose what was happening to her mother, who had not believed her. Her father was no longer in contact, and she was an only child. At school, she had a sense of differentness owing to her family not fitting the conventional heterosexual couple and owing to the fact she did not have a father and siblings included in her family. As a consequence, she had felt an outsider at school and had not been able to settle enough into relationships with teachers and classmates to achieve either socially or academically. This then meant her career choices were limited more to blue-collar careers, which she bored of easily and did not engage with. Her employment as a check-out operator at a local supermarket had ended after a dispute with her line manager, resulting in her walking off the job without any further contact. These interpersonal outbursts seemed to be a wider theme of her adult life, limiting her opportunities for having relationship, financial and employment stability. The turmoil in her present life was perhaps enough to address without the exploration of issues from the past.

After she had been introduced to the self-help guide *The Courage to Heal* (Bass & Davis, 1988), Fiona remembered more of what had been regular sexual abuse from her stepmother from the age of 12 years through to when she was 16 years old. She was confused about her sexuality as she realised by high school that she had been sexually abused by her stepmother. She had avoided all romantic and sexual advances at high school and up to the present time.

After seeing me fortnightly for three months, she asked that I assist her to lodge a sensitive claim for compensation for her abuse through the publicly funded no-faults scheme offered by the New Zealand government under the Accident Compensation and Rehabilitation Corporation. In supervision with the team, the team members advised this might be a broader part of her healing, as Fiona was hoping to gain the deposit on her first home with the monies of her compensation. Her intention in lodging a sensitive claim and applying for financial compensation for what had occurred with her stepmother was to 'start a new life' free from memories of the past.

We completed the report required in the application for her sensitive claim in our sessions, and I explained that a consent form for the release of information to the ACC was needed for the purposes of establishing her sensitive claim for cover. After this explanation, she agreed to sign this consent for the release of information to the ACC. Fiona thanked me for my help and, in passing, she remarked that I had 'light blue eyes' that were 'like my stepmother's'. Interestingly, I have hazel eyes, but the projection of characteristics of the perpetrator of her abuse on to me was evident in her comment. I did not realise this at the time, but she dropped out of contact due to disclosing details of her abuse to me too early in the contact. This may have evoked a shame response. Paradoxically, she felt safe enough to project on to me characteristics of her perpetrator, which was deeply troubling to me in retrospect, though, for Herman (1992) and the New Trauma therapists, this was a predictable part of our contact.

I heard by letter from the ACC that Fiona's sensitive claim for cover for future treatment costs in relation to medical and counselling care had been successful. Second, she had been awarded NZ$10,000 by the ACC in recognition of the mental injury she had sustained as a teenager inflicted by a trusted parental figure.

I was pleased to hear that the new start she wanted for her life might now be within her grasp. However, I felt a sense of confusion about the impact of raising her early trauma and whether it had been 'too much and too soon'. An alternative view I considered is that perhaps therapy and healing from past trauma are not the goals of all women who present for help at our clinic. Third, I wondered if I had done harm by raising all of the details of her abuse which, at first, had been something we had contracted to do in our sessions. I was left puzzled by the request for claim and compensation and, in retrospect, I wondered if this was the sole importance of our contact from Fiona's perspective. If that was the underlying reason for referral, disclosure had a more practical than therapeutic aim and function from her perspective.

The implications for working with women survivors of CSA who choose to disclose historical issues in a current crisis

The key difference between the classical Freudian conceptualisation of the stages of psychoanalysis and the stages of healing in the New Trauma Therapy is the view that the survivor is the initiator of the contact and the process, which may or may not include disclosure. The practitioner, under more humanistic understandings of trauma, resilience and recovery for women CSA survivors, is a co-learner and collaborator in the client's process. Practitioners provide a crucible within which the woman client moves through the stages of recovery in a spiralling backwards and forwards rather than in a linear pattern. Therefore, ruptures and withdrawal are part of the process, leading to 'stop-start' moments in the contact. Briere (1996) endorses the need for the therapist to move at the client's pace, paying attention to honouring the coping strategies developed at each stage of the healing from CSA.

The case study of Fiona illustrates the dangers of moving too quickly from a therapeutic role to a forensic one, which was required to complete the supporting report for her claim for cover for treatment expenses and compensation. Guided by a self-help approach in which the client had defined her goals, I had contracted to develop the ACC assessment based on her wishes. However, we had only established the safety with insufficient scaffolding for the remembering process. Knowing what I now know, I realise that this is a common 'rookie error' for those who are new to a field of practice (I was only two years post qualifying with my Master's in social work) and for whom believing in the client's account was the priority. The necessity for probing questions on the nature, duration and relationship with the perpetrator had transformed my role in our relationship from that of collaborator to the top–down 'expert-knows-best'. The New Trauma Therapy had suggested that the relationship in which there is a mutual search for meaning from the client's perspective differs from this role of assessor for a public insurance authority. This approach, in which disclosure is met with support and belief, can be undermined if the contents of disclosure are used for other purposes beyond the clinic. If disclosure had been met with disbelief by trusted figures, such as Fiona had experienced with her mother, the perilous nature of the other's response to her attempt to tell again is likely in itself to be traumatic for the client and to trigger a re-experiencing of the original denial during the last disclosure. Therapists, therefore, need to delay any insurance work for claim cover until the grieving and mourning phase for the childhood the woman feels deprived of is completed (Herman, 1992).

Having the availability of a clinical supervisory relationship was also somewhat lacking earlier in my career in mental health. My team leader, who was responsible for my clinical supervision, was a social worker who was not trained in psychodynamic psychotherapy. Because of her background, she did not see or understand the complexities of traumatic transference and countertransference. Nor was there any framework for understanding the potential for vicarious traumatisation. Both secondary trauma and vicarious traumatisation will be discussed in forthcoming chapters. The main forum for discussing cases in our community mental health clinic during the time I worked with Fiona was a weekly group supervision group in which individual practitioners discussed their cases within the multidisciplinary team. We would discuss what the focus was with each client on our caseload in an assessment and treatment planning model of peer review.

On the positive side, Fiona was successful in having her sensitive claim accepted on the basis of her application and the report we compiled together. She was successful in obtaining cover of all future therapy costs related to her sexual abuse trauma and the mental injury caused by these events involving her step-parent. She also obtained financial compensation that might change her life by providing options for homeownership goals.

Further reflections on the case

Attachment, when disrupted in childhood owing to childhood sexual abuse, leading to betrayals of trust during adulthood makes the task of forging and maintaining the therapeutic relationship difficult and complicated. There are perils and pitfalls that those new to the field will likely find confusing and deeply troubling in this process. When material and experiences from the past related to the original abuse arise and are disowned by the client, through the process of projection, there are key moments in which the therapist may become the abuser without realising what is occurring between them and the client. Therefore, the powerful feelings evoked by the transference between client and professional can be traumatic for the helping professional and require a skilled clinical supervisor to successfully navigate the relationship.

The models of clinical supervision that are considered to be helpful when counselling professionals are dealing with such complex issues as childhood sexual abuse are relational in nature. There is also a holistic focus needed on both the personal and the professional issues arising from working with traumatic disclosures (Pack, 2009). As trauma impacts the whole self of the therapist, and the use of self is central in therapeutic endeavour with adult survivors, knowing oneself and one's biography is also central to handling the disclosure of abuse so that disruption to the therapeutic relationship is minimised.

The styles of clinical supervision of practice that allow for the counsellor to explore and discuss the impact of seeing the client in terms of how the process and content are affecting them and the feelings that are evoked are all matters considered to be important (Pack, 2011). Assessing the potential for parallel processes occurring between the client and the therapist, including vicarious traumatisation, is also important when dealing with traumatic disclosures. As the case of Fiona illustrates, building self-awareness in the practitioner role through clinical critique and review with a trusted peer or peer group is much recommended to address these transferences and parallel processes.

Conclusion

Knowledge, when working within Freudian psychoanalysis and psychotherapy pre the 1960s, was still considered the preserve of the scientist who tests theory within a predominantly logocentric paradigm. However, for more recent developments in theory formation, prompted by the needs of returning veterans and women's rights, there has been a changed context due to the historical times and the challenges raised for the status quo. In the field of working with women survivors of CSA and the disclosures that were made around the time of the burgeoning feminist movement, self-help guides came out of a change of ideological positioning where women were encouraged to drive the content and process of their therapy. In the field of psychotherapy and other helping professions, the predominant theoretical concepts underpinning practice have been critiqued in favour of a more socially constructed vision of social reality. The therapeutic relationship has itself become reformulated in this revision. Unlike the traditional psychoanalytic tradition, where the therapist carefully controlled what happened in the therapy room and represented the 'blank screen' on to which the client projected through a process of free association, a mutual search for meaning was embarked upon. This collaborative search for answers is intrinsic to the relationship between client and practitioner (Kahn, 1991). It is the therapeutic relationship so reformulated that facilitates disclosure at the client's pace, and it incorporates all past experiences of disclosure. This cautions practitioners working with women who are survivors of CSA to look at theories of practice that equip them to understand the importance of this quality of relationship. The New Trauma therapists were central to making this paradigm shift towards an understanding of the fact that treatment on the basis of diagnosis and intervention has failed many women survivors of CSA (Herman, 1992; Courtois, 1997). This reconceptualisation of the importance of a relationship that is collaborative, paced and staged more accurately fits the work of helping practitioners who work with women sexual abuse survivors who have been multiply abused and oppressed.

In the next chapter, we move to explore the importance of narrative and narrative theory guiding practitioners to provide women survivors of CSA with the opportunity to tell their personal narratives in their own voice, across the lifespan. The importance of narrative is another development in the trauma-informed and recovery literature for women survivors of CSA who face decisions about disclosure.

References

Alaggia, R. (2004). Many ways of telling: expanding conceptualizations of child sexual abuse disclosure. *Child Abuse and Neglect*, 28, 1213–1227.

American Psychiatric Association. (2013). *Diagnostic and Statistical Manual of Mental Disorders* (5th ed.). American Psychiatric Association.

Bass, E., & Davis, L. (1988). *The Courage to Heal* (1st ed.). Harper Perennial.

Bass, E., & Davis, L. (1992). *The Courage to Heal* (3rd ed.). Harper Perennial.

Becker, K. D., Stuewig, J., & McCloskey, L. A. (2010). Traumatic stress symptoms of women exposed to different forms of childhood victimization and intimate partner violence. *Journal of Interpersonal Violence*, 25(9), 1699–1715. doi:10.1177/0886260509354578

Bennett, C. (2018). Moment of reckoning. *Next Magazine*, 37–41.

Boston Women's Health Book Collective. (1976). *Our Bodies, Ourselves: A Book by and for Women*. Simon & Schuster.

Bottoms, B. L., Peter-Hagene, L. C., Epstein, M. A., Wiley, T. R., Reynolds, C. E., & Rudnicki, A. G. (2014). Abuse characteristics and individual differences related to disclosing childhood sexual, physical, and emotional abuse and witnessed domestic violence. *Journal of Interpersonal Violence*, 31(7), 1308–1339. doi:10.1177/0886260514564155

Brazelton, J. F. (2015). The secret storm: exploring the disclosure process of African American women survivors of child sexual abuse across the life course. *Traumatology*, 21(3), 181.

Briere, J. (1989). *Therapy for Adults Molested as Children: Beyond Survival.* Springer.

Briere, J. (1996). *Therapy for Adults Molested as Children: Beyond Survival.* Springer.

Courtois, C. (1988). *Healing the Incest Wound: Adult Survivors in Therapy.* W.W. Norton. Courtois, C. A. (1997). Healing the incest wound: a treatment update with attention to recovered-memory issues. *American Journal of Psychotherapy*, 51(4), 464–496. doi:10.1176/appi.psychotherapy.1997.51.4.464

Dalenberg, C. J. (2000). *Countertransference and the Treatment of Trauma.* American Psychological Association.

Domhardt, M., Münzer, A., Fegert, J. M., & Goldbeck, L. (2015). Resilience in survivors of child sexual abuse: a systematic review of the literature. *Trauma Violence Abuse*, 16(4), 476–493. doi:10.1177/1524838014557288

Freud, S. (1909). Five lectures on psycho-analysis. *SE*, 11.

Gasker, J. A. (1999). *I Never Told Anyone This Before: Managing the Initial Disclosure of Sexual Abuse Re-Collections.* Psychology Press.

Giacci, E., Straits, K. J., Gelman, A., Miller-Walfish, S., Iwuanyanwu, R., & Miller, E. (2022). Intimate partner and sexual violence, reproductive coercion, and reproductive health among American Indian and Alaska native women: a narrative interview study. *Journal of Women's Health*, 31(1), 13–22.

Gilligan, C. (1982). *In a Different Voice: Psychological Theory and Women's Development.* Harvard University Press.

Glover, D. A., Loeb, T. B., Carmona, J. V., Sciolla, A., Zhang, M., Myers, H. F., & Wyatt, G. E. (2010). Childhood sexual abuse severity and disclosure predict post-traumatic stress symptoms and biomarkers in ethnic minority women. *Journal of Trauma and Dissociation*, 11(2), 152–173.

Gupta, S., Bonanno, G. A., Noll, J. G., Putnam, F. W., Keltner, D., & Trickett, P. K. (2011). Anger expression and adaptation to childhood sexual abuse: the role of disclosure. *Psychological Trauma: Theory, Research, Practice, and Policy*, 3(2), 171.

Herman, J. (1992). *Trauma and Recovery.* Basic Books.

Jeremiah, R. D., Quinn, C. R., & Alexis, J. M. (2017). Exposing the culture of silence: inhibiting factors in the prevention, treatment, and mitigation of sexual abuse in the Eastern Caribbean. *Child Abuse and Neglect*, 66, 53–63. doi:10.1016/j.chiabu.2017.01.029

Kahn, M. (1991). *Between Therapist and Client: The New Relationship.* Macmillan.

Lahav, Y., & Elklit, A. (2016). The cycle of healing – dissociation and attachment during treatment of CSA survivors. *Child Abuse and Neglect*, 60, 67–76. doi:10.1016/j.chiabu.2016.09.009

McElvaney, R. (2015). Disclosure of child sexual abuse: delays, non-disclosure and partial disclosure. What the research tells us and implications for practice. *Child Abuse Review*, 24(3), 159–169. doi:10.1002/car.2280

Ministry of Justice, New Zealand. (1961). Crimes Act 1961.

Pack, M. (2009). Supervision as a liminal space: towards a dialogic relationship. *Gestalt Journal of Australia and New Zealand*, 5(2), 60–78.

Pack, M. (2011). Defining moments in practice. Clinical supervision as a method of promoting critical reflection in fieldwork: a qualitative inquiry. *Aotearoa New Zealand Social Work*, 23(4), 45–54.

Pack, M. (2016). *Self-Help for Trauma Therapists: A Practitioner's Guide.* Routledge.

Rogers, C. (1995). *On Becoming a Person: A Therapist's View of Psychotherapy.* Houghton Mifflin Harcourt.

Rueda, P., Ferragut, M., Cerezo, M. V., & Ortiz-Tallo, M. (2021). Child sexual abuse in Mexican women: type of experience, age, perpetrator, and disclosure. *International Journal of Environmental Research and Public Health*, 18(13). doi:10.3390/ijerph18136931

Simmel, C., Postmus, J. L., & Lee, I. (2012). Sexual revictimization in adult women: examining factors associated with their childhood and adulthood experiences. *Journal of Child Sexual Abuse*, 21(5), 593–611. doi:10.1080/10538712.2012.690836

Van der Kolk, B. A., McFarlane, A. C., & Weisaeth, L. (Eds.). (1996). *Traumatic Stress: The Effects of Overwhelming Experience on Mind, Body, and Society.* Guilford Press.

Wallis, C. R. D., & Woodworth, M. (2021). Non-offending caregiver support in cases of child sexual abuse: an examination of the impact of support on formal disclosures. *Child Abuse and Neglect*, 113. doi:10.1016/j.chiabu.2021.104929

World Health Organization (WHO). (2017). Guidelines for medico-legal care for victims of sexual violence. Retrieved 11 November from www.who.int/violence injury prevention/resources/publications/en/guidelines

2 Disclosure and the importance of narrative across the life course

> I said no. Repeatedly. He didn't stop. I had felt so pretty in my first formal ball dress. Not so pretty when he pushed me up against a car and grappled with the fabric. Not so pretty afterwards on my hands and knees vomiting, yet unable to rid myself of the sick feeling that engulfed me. Not so pretty in the days and weeks that followed, as I took refuge in the school toilets from the whispers of 'slag' that echoed around my sixth form.
>
> (Cath Bennett, journalist, writing of her experience of being sexually assaulted as an adolescent in her research article 'Moment of Reckoning', in *Next Magazine*, December 2018, p. 37)

Introduction

In this chapter, narrative and storytelling are reflected on in relation to the disclosure of CSA by women. Speaking or writing about one's abuse provides a context for healing for women who are survivors of CSA. As the above example of disclosure illustrates, there is a wider social context surrounding sexual abuse. These milestones in life are remembered as part of the fabric of one's life and are witnessed by others, alongside memories of CSA. In this way, journalist Cath Bennett writes of the idealism, naïveté and rite of passage of the school formal underpinning her personal narrative of a date rape as a 17 year old. This night, expected to be a happy time of celebration, changed her life in adulthood. Her narrative above acknowledges the abuse along with a night filled with high hopes for the future. Her optimism was suddenly transformed into a nightmare surrounded by emotional pain and shaming by her peers. Her teenage friends and fellow classmates, in their naïveté, assumed the version of events recounted to be consensual sex rather than the reality of a violent rape.

Helping professionals are often the first people women survivors of CSA disclose to, making them the first witnesses to the shards and fragments of traumatic memories, witnessed often in first-time telling. Disclosure is often made retrospectively, in adulthood, which is a kind of reminiscing about a time now remote from the life stage in which the original abuse occurred, as Cath Bennett's (2018) recollections of her own abuse at the school formal as a teenager illustrate. Now a successful journalist, in a happy, committed

DOI: 10.4324/9781032669205-2

partnership and mother of three sons, she reflects from the vantage point of an adult woman, wondering about the many ways in which the incident could have impacted her identity had it not been for the many protective factors present in her life at the time of her abuse and currently. She continues with reflections of how she tackled her own and society's negative beliefs about the rape and revises her self-blame as a teenager by redirecting responsibility for what happened to the perpetrator of her abuse:

> I haven't let my experience as a 17 year old define me. For many years I believed I brought it on myself – I was drunk, probably flirtatious, I followed him outside, I didn't try hard enough to fight him off – but I gradually came to realise it wasn't my fault.
>
> (Bennett, 2018, p. 41)

In this example, disclosure of CSA happened in relation to others; it is an interpersonal process that can mirror the abuse itself, as the previous chapter and the case study of Fiona illustrated. Often, there is a need to tell the story involving both the societal narrative alongside the individual story of what happened. Part of the survivor's story includes what the ongoing legacy of the abuse has been throughout their life. These accounts most frequently happen retrospectively, from a position of comparative safety as an adult.

How women tell to another: their experiences of disclosure

Fragments of experience of CSA are often remembered by adult survivors as disjointed flashbacks. This is owing to the nature of traumatic memory, which is processed in part of the brain responsible for primal 'fight and flight' responses (van der Kolk et al., 1996). Relationship and connectedness with the survivor are the paramount considerations in the process of healing from CSA. As we saw in the previous chapter, drawing from the New Trauma Therapy, traumatised clients report dissatisfaction in therapy when their sense of the relationship with their therapist fails to meet their emotional need for connection adequately (Dalenberg, 2000). This reformulated therapeutic relationship was part of the revision initiated by the theorising of the New Trauma therapists (Briere, 1996; Courtois, 1997; Herman, 1992). Within this reconceptualisation, the 'blank screen' or 'expert-knows-best' approaches are considered to be unhelpful as they can further traumatise rather than assist the adult survivor of CSA. These dissatisfactions from clients are most often related to the accuracy of the helping professional's reading of the client's emotional cues and the congruence of their response. Without emotional engagement and congruence, the dissatisfied client may see the helping practitioner as failing to provide the 'safe' therapeutic environment crucial to the healing process. Narrative is a means by which therapists make sense of how the woman survivor has been impacted at each life stage and so fosters engagement in the unfolding story of the woman's life as a lived experience.

Findings from the research literature illuminate ways by which the initial act of disclosing/telling does not necessarily result in healing from CSA. Instead, the research suggests that the pathway to healing extends long past the initial experience of disclosure and the content of what is told. How the story of CSA is recounted to another alters over the life course as an understanding of the enormity of what happened grows with age and maturity (Mooney & McGregor, 2018). This ongoing nature of disclosure is in part because of the changes that occur in the stories we tell ourselves about what has happened. This inner dialogue, in turn, changes the stories we tell and retell others. It is essential, therefore, for women to engage in acknowledgement of and reconciliation to the sexual abuse over time, and often across the life course. Positive relationships with partners and parents and functioning in their community and family support the ongoing need for women to rework and reframe their abuse experiences as a lived experience across time (Brazelton, 2015a; Brazelton, 2015b). Gasker (1999, p. 24) concurs with this view and writes of the therapist's role in disclosure as validating a client's account of what happened earlier in life while bracketing or suspending judgement about the historical accuracy of the events. Within a narrative, life course perspective, one adapts to the changing individual and social conditions of one's life, providing a continuity of experience for the individual. For example, Salzberg (2017), an authority on Buddhist compassion and insight practices and an internationally acclaimed meditation teacher, in her research with key advisors who have been on their own healing journeys from trauma, recounts how one's own narrative can be told in different ways depending on the development of awareness about one's life, including the intangible or spiritual dimensions of life. During an interview with Salzberg, her friend and fellow author Barbara Graham reflects on what occurred with a trusted camp counsellor when she was a 14 year old. As a 44 year old, Graham realised this to have been sexual abuse. Her understanding of this trusted other's behaviour was unavailable to her as a teenager:

> It took me thirty years to understand that what took place between my camp counsellor and me the summer I was fourteen – and she was twenty-eight – was sexual abuse. It took me another decade for me to forgive her for touching me and – hardest of all – to stop blaming myself … When at last I understood what happened, I was stricken by a grief that had been there all along but which I never knew I carried.
>
> (Salzberg, 2017, p. 51)

Knowing that a trusted other's behaviour was sexual abuse sometimes comes as a discovery in adulthood. Looking back at one's childhood prompts new insights. The subsequent recounting of events often changes the survivor's interpretation of events and so the substance of one's life story. This revised or new narrative can lead to further insights that are then available to be integrated into the revised personal narrative in new and often surprising ways, in an interactive and cyclical fashion over time.

The transformational potential of disclosure and of retelling of one's life story is at the core of narrative theory on which narrative therapy is based. One of the most formative influences of modern narrative theory has been the founding theorising of Michael White and David Epston working from the Dulwich Centre in Adelaide, Australia. Like the influence of the New Trauma Therapy on present-day understanding of trauma-informed theory, the concept of telling one's story as being formative of the self and identity represents a paradigm shift from earlier understandings of the 'expert-knows-best' approaches, beginning with Freudian psychoanalysis and the free association that provided the material for the expert to analyse. The value of storytelling is predicated on the idea that understanding the processes of rebuilding the self can be facilitated through an iterative process of disclosure in the context of one's wider life trajectory.

The role of disclosure and narrative from a life course perspective

Narrative therapy is defined by White (1995) and Epston and White (1992) as a process by which therapists work alongside their clients to identify ways of discussing their lives that contribute to a sense of 'personal agency'. The goal of sexual abuse recovery from a narrative theoretical positioning is seen as restoring power to the survivor's sense of autonomy. This personal autonomy derives from the experience of being an authority on, and an author of, one's life.

> Helping professionals draw distinctions about the ways of speaking about the self that contribute to experiences of being affirmed and also those ways of speaking that lead to a sense of isolation or marginalisation. There are discourses and stories that subtract from a sense of personal agency and that undermine an appreciation of one's authoritativeness.
>
> (White, 1995, pp. 121–122)

The idea that women survivors of CSA can become enmeshed in the problem-defined stories they tell about themselves, or that others tell about them, can detract from this sense of personal agency and being an authority on one's life. Cath Bennett's disclosure to her teenage peers, for a period of her life, made her actions rather than the perpetrator's 'the problem' (Bennett, 2018).

The narrative theory concept of 'externalising the problem' (White & Epston, 1990, p. 30) shares much in common with postmodern thinking about the deconstruction of language to reveal the underlying import or 'taken-for-granted' meaning of our everyday life. Meaning in this broader view is derived from what has been termed 'lived experience' within narrative theory (White, 1995, citing Geertz, 1975). It is the lived experience that is the focus of new directions in research on disclosure of CSA which I will connect to narrative theorising in this chapter.

'Re-authoring' personal narratives in 'liminal spaces'

Beyond the concept of being the author of one's life, the notion of 're-authoring' has relevance to the disclosure of CSA (White, 1995). The concept of re-authoring used by narrative theorists such as White (1995) derives from Barbara Myerhoff, a cultural anthropologist who observed and participated with elders in a community centre in her local Jewish community in Florida, USA. Her ethnographic research aimed to observe the lived experiences of Jewish elders who were in the process of making a new life in America. While undertaking ethnographic study, she developed the concept of 're-authoring', informed by the founding work of cultural anthropologist Victor Turner (Myerhoff, 1982). 'Re-authoring' one's life describes the sense of disjuncture that her research participants, who were Jewish elders, experienced in migrating to and living in America after enduring the horrors of the Holocaust in Nazi-dominated Europe. Myerhoff draws from the extended narratives of Jewish elders to describe the ways in which they tell and retell their personal biographies to encompass the experience of trauma, from the position of safety, having come to a new life in America (Myerhoff, 1982). Their accounts are overlaid with the traditions, stories, language and ritual from the 'old country' of war-torn Europe. In the telling and retelling of their stories, she notes that a 're-membering' takes place for the teller. Friends and family, once lost in time and place, are reunited with their authors in the storytelling process. New life-enhancing possibilities are created in personal narrative by this process of remembering.

Narrative therapy's theoretical perspective is one that assumes that every individual is the author of their life, with the power and autonomy to change their narrative by the way the life story is told and retold. Within each life stage, a process of 're-authoring' occurs to integrate aspects of life that are prominent within that phase. Concurrently, there is an impetus to synthesise learning associated with these life transitions as being connected with earlier life experiences (White & Epston, 1990). Narrative theory offers a useful paradigm for working with women survivors' disclosures as, within this theoretical framework, the life narrative is considered to be the creator of the self, and, conversely, the self shapes the survivor's life narrative interactively (Gasker, 1999, p. 34). This paradigm shift from expert-knows-best to the woman survivor being the authority on her life is a radical reconceptualisation. For example, Gasker (1999), in her research on group therapy with women survivors of CSA, found that the participants in the group therapy she was observing needed to establish safety within their support group before they could feel there was the emotional safety present among group members to be able to disclose. Once they felt 'safe', she noted that the timing of the disclosure was important in the group process as the opportunity was seen at a time when the participants had developed relationships of trust with one another and with the group facilitator. One of the participants disclosed her recollections of CSA almost in passing, in a conversation following a coffee break, which prompted other group members to disclose details of their abuse during childhood. These disclosures were completely unprompted by the group facilitator. The focus of the group was to act as a support network to assist women coping with mental health issues and with their daily lives in the present. All members who disclosed CSA during this one session over the coffee break told the facilitator that that chat in the coffee break among the group members was enough to raise the issue of CSA in a general way within the group. Following this discussion, they expressed a wish as individuals to 'move on' to explore how the abuse experience had impacted their current lives, rather than dwelling on the details of what happened in the past. Gasker's recommendation is to assist survivors to integrate historical abuse experiences in the present by giving the women survivors in the group the power to choose when and how to disclose matters related to CSA:

> The first step, then in recognising the power of authorship in one's own life story is the experience of telling it in a safe environment. The next step is recognising that one might be a competent author. Evidence of this recognition may be the movement of the traumatic story to the context of the current events. When the life story is focused on the present, it necessarily takes on a dynamic aspect in which the teller alters it to suit the environment and the audience.
>
> (Gasker, 1999, p. 52)

Different life events present the need to integrate the past with the present to make sense of, and to learn to cope with, the current challenge. For example, a current life narrative involving the diagnosis of a woman survivor of CSA as being unable to conceive and/or give birth to a healthy baby can put strains on relationships owing to negative social status being associated with childlessness. Persistent attempts to conceive using reproductive technologies may retrigger feelings of anger, helplessness and powerlessness formerly associated with historical abuse. Similarly, entering a new relationship or a new course of study, a health concern later in life, redundancy and job change can all be associated with experiences of stress and involve issues relating to a lack of power over one's life, prompted by change and involving present and historical grief and loss. All of these events present a need to evolve new life narratives to explain the past and to move forward. The abuse narrative from the past may be revisited as some reformulation of identity is necessitated by the particular life event or transition, as I have found in my clinical experience over the last 30 years.

Some of the themes in the disclosure of CSA by women are usefully informed by narrative theory. These concepts include: first-time disclosures, epiphany moments, re-authoring and liminal spaces, which I will move on to discuss. Connections with life course theory will be made before these themes are illustrated with a case study.

First-time disclosures

The first-time telling of one's life narrative as it relates to CSA for adult women has a special therapeutic importance as, in the choice point about whether to disclose or not, the client risks rejection, disbelief and invalidation in the initial attempt. As we saw in the previous chapter, if the client has been traumatised by a trusted adult disbelieving what was said or minimising their experiences, in this rejection there can be a sense of betrayal for the woman. If the original CSA is in the context of the adult woman having been abandoned or rejected by an inconsistent caregiver, the response of the practitioner to a client's disclosure of CSA can make or break the therapeutic relationship. As the case study in Chapter One suggests, moving into a forensic assessment for the details of what happened too soon can risk re-traumatising the client and prompt dropout or an early 'flight into wellness'.

Hearing the woman survivor's first disclosure of CSA can be a powerful, and at times, troubling experience for the helping professional. The notion of witnessing the historical injustice that has remained silent for so long can bring with it a sense of outrage that requires ongoing clinical supervision and case consultation for the practitioner to deal with the traumatic transferences that can arise. In forthcoming chapters, we will explore more of the practitioner's responses to disclosure including the potential for vicarious traumatisation in the case studies presented (Pearlman & Saakvitne, 1995).

A moment of insight

Some narrative theorists describe the recollection of CSA by adult survivors as being an 'epiphany experience' that becomes prominent in the life narrative at any one point in time (Gasker, 1999, p. 31). These experiences are conceptualised as 'high points', 'low points' or 'turning points' in the woman's journey through life (Gasker, 1999, p. 31). These events may not be seen as significant by the survivor when they occur, but rather something about them becomes out of sync with the self-image held by the individual. This dissonance with their concept of who they are prompts the need to reassess and redefine their identity and relationships with others. Thus, recognising the ongoing impact of CSA can be an example of an epiphany experience (Gasker, 1999, p. 31). If disclosure happens across a lifetime during key moments of insight, disclosure of CSA comes to be seen as a more fluid, interactive and dynamic process where alternative versions of the self may be brought to therapy depending on what is happening in one's everyday life.

While the New Trauma therapists would define episodes of dissociation where fragments of one's traumatic past intrude into one's current life, narrative theory reframes dissociation as 'disintegrated recollections' (Gasker, 1999, p. 36). These recollections may have been disclosed to another or not and may cause some form of crisis when remembered. A characteristic of disintegrated recollections, which may come in the guise of flashbacks or nightmares, is that they can be experienced in a host of different ways. In my experience, there is often a sense of being at a crossroads, or at a choice point in one's life, where the former life needs to change in some way or relationships need to change to accommodate new understandings that the survivor is developing about her life in whatever phase of life she is in currently. The client may feel out of kilter with her current life. The goal of therapy may be in terms of integration of the new memory, fitting an experience into her existing life narrative so that it becomes congruent with her self-image. Therefore, a life narrative that acknowledges and incorporates the experience of CSA into a woman survivor's narrative is the major goal of contact with a helping professional when dissonance is experienced.

The importance of 're-authoring'

The role of the narrative therapist is as a 'witness' (Herman, 1992) and a collaborator in finding the redefined identity and life narrative. This is where the notion of the therapist supporting clients to 're-author' becomes central to healing from CSA for adult women. As White and Epston (1990) theorise, the functional story of one's life incorporates the past and one's significant others in the present in a dynamic and creative re-storying of one's life within a community of relationships.

Furthermore White and Epston suggest that women can become enmeshed by and within 'dominant discourses' which are endorsed by powerful groups in society. Such enmeshment can disrupt the woman survivor's sense of 'personal agency' (Epston & White, 1992; White, 1995; White & Epston, 1990). When such a disjuncture exists, there is a choice point for women survivors to present for help (White, 1995). The point of the woman choosing to disclose her personal narrative about historical CSA is to listen to that narrative which has become marginalised through having being silenced. This marginalised narrative may exist uneasily alongside the predominant societal narrative. The task of therapy is to acknowledge that these narratives have become marginalised by the prevailing societal narratives. The act of listening and engaging with marginalised narratives is an act of reparation, implying that both narratives exist, albeit uneasily, alongside one another and are each constitutive of different but related worlds within which the survivor of CSA functions (White & Epston, 1990).

Liminal spaces

Associated with the notion of re-authoring and marginalised narratives that exist within the predominant or societal narrative, there is the concept of 'liminal space'. The concept of liminality is derived from the work of Barbara Myerhoff (1982) who, in turn, developed the concept from another cultural anthropologist, Victor Turner. Myerhoff, drawing on Turner's model, sees liminality as a stage in one's life that is noteworthy as a 'rite of passage' that offers a pause for reflection. The stories told by the Jewish women elders in the community studied by Myerhoff explained how their past trauma was healed by the sharing of stories about escaping the Holocaust in Europe during World War Two. Second, she discovered the sharing of new narratives by Jewish elders about how they made a new life in America was constitutive of new narratives in the present. In the various iterations involved in the telling and retelling of these narratives, she conceptualises this disclosure process as existing in what she termed a 'liminal space' (Myerhoff, 1982). This is a place of transition, between the new life and the old, that exists not in one or the other, but between the two realms of past and present. Paradoxically, both iterations can exist as if in a parallel universe, with the past trauma explored from the safety of the new life. Liminal spaces, therefore, are seen as being conceptually transitional zones between the 'known and the unknown'. This is the conceptual space between arrival and departure, which is neither, but exists between the two. It involves the major storylines of the person, the subplots that remain untold or minimised and that exist in the wider family and societal discourses that surround the woman survivor.

As such, 'liminal spaces', in which Myerhoff conceptualised that the Jewish elder women's experience exists, are places of promise and possibility, peril and danger. Women's experience, generally, is seen by Myerhoff as existing on the margin and periphery, not fitting the world of men and of mainstream patriarchal society but, rather, standing outside it, to be viewed on its own terms. Being Jewish female elders in North American middle-class society, she reflects, further positions her women participants on the outer fringes of mainstream society. By validating their stories in the presence of the other Jewish women who attend the community centre, Myerhoff brings their experience 'back into being' in new and life-renewing ways. In so doing, Myerhoff uses narrative that transcends notions of power within the predominant discourse of white North American middle-class society.

Myerhoff's concept of liminality offers an explanation of the ways in which women exist in a patriarchal world while maintaining their own narrative as women within the prevailing societal narrative that is male-dominated. The site of therapy could also be considered a site of liminality. It is a pause in the everyday life context from which an individual is invited and supported when women survivors are deliberating on past CSA and its effects upon them.

For women survivors of CSA, this liminal space offers sanctuary and an opportunity to deliberate on the impact of CSA in an ongoing supportive relationship. Within that extended reflective process with a counsellor or therapist, the decision about whether to tell and retell one's personal story as a springboard for creating another iteration of what happened with the CSA can be explored from a position of safety. In her autobiographical memoir, Leibrich (2015) describes her lifelong search for 'sanctuary' that is closely associated with finding a spiritual retreat from the vicissitudes of life. Reflecting upon her earlier life and the difficulties in her adult relationship, in which she felt betrayed, she describes finding 'a place in her heart' that was there throughout her life but remained invisible, awaiting discovery. Her memoir was written seven years before her death. In her late 60s, she had new insights about past trauma in her life offered by her later years (Leibrich, 2015). This kind of discovery is at the heart of a life course perspective, which we will now explore.

The life course perspective

Universally, there are certain life events and developmental phases that have been found to prompt a revisiting of one's personal narrative. The life course model details the range of junctures that are related to different life transitions and developmental phases. Diverse cultural values are associated with these differing life changes that occur for women and align with this life course model. Some of these forks in the road involve biological changes, and others are based on the notion of social and cultural rites of passage or milestones achieved through development and maturation. Such rites of passage, therefore, include some of the following life themes (not in any sequential order): reaching puberty; entering a relationship or partnering; graduating from a course of study and transitioning into a career; first sexual experiences; pregnancy; giving birth; separating from a relationship or maturing into the same, or another, relationship; menopause; retirement; and getting older. Ultimately, in approaching ageing, there may be a sense of the loss of youth and a preparation for death (Gitterman & Germain, 2008, p. 191). Health concerns, including how to manage fertility, what happens when a pregnancy occurs, menopause and ageing, illness and dying, are all universally understood life transitions which have psychological, socio-cultural and emotional aspects associated with them (Gitterman & Germain, 2008, p. 191).

In terms of challenges for women survivors of CSA, recent studies on the legacy of CSA for women have shown specific impacts affecting the whole of life, including choice of partner and intimate partner violence (IPV), attainment of education and employment, mental health vulnerabilities, ongoing anxiety about sex and insomnia. These research findings, therefore, need to be factored into an understanding of how to deal with CSA in an ongoing way with women survivors of CSA.

Superimposing the template of the life course perspective over a life that has been affected by a history of CSA suggests the importance of having opportunities for reflection in liminal spaces. I conceptualise the liminal space as representing the space between disclosure or revisiting the legacy of CSA and its original storyline, alongside the current life challenge relating to the life trajectory. It is as though the current life event triggers a reiteration of the original CSA impact, and, with the remembering, the original abuse narrative may arise again. This conceptual model aligns with the literature on the long-term legacy of childhood trauma for women survivors of CSA. This ongoing impact includes effects on mental health, sleep, choice of partner and adult relationships, sexuality and decisions around whether to become a parent. Using longitudinal research designs provides a liminal space for women survivors to tell and retell researchers about their lived experience of CSA over time.

The long-term legacy of CSA for women across the life course

Histories of CSA have an enduring impact on women's life choices and life course, with a connection between CSA and later mental health issues (Becker et al., 2010, p. 1710). This study aligns with other research studies finding lifelong issues for women's psychological well-being when they disclose details of their CSA and are not believed. The long-lasting effects of CSA throughout adulthood suggest that it is imperative that professionals identify and treat CSA for the future well-being of the next generation, in terms of adult women survivor's children as they progress into adolescence and adulthood, as there is a need to promote their mental health through gaps and difficulties in parenting. Careful assessment and early intervention/treatment are needed to avoid the risks of later impeding their children's or adolescents' lives through exposure to mental health conditions, as has been documented in the literature. For example, IPV has been studied extensively with adult women survivors of CSA (Easton et al., 2011). The conclusion from such studies is that there is often an increased likelihood of subsequent abuse in adult relationships when there is no working model of what a safe relationship or parent is. Becker et al. (2010) acknowledge that not all women survivors of CSA enter subsequent treatment for IPV, but practitioners need to be aware of how the dynamics of CSA may function to place adult women at risk, throughout the life course, of subsequent abuse in their adult relationships. Discussing women survivors' narratives may illuminate how the underlying interpersonal dynamics of subsequent intimate relationships have operated across the lifespan to place women at risk and help to buffer the more negative legacy of CSA. Similarly, Zamir and Lavee (2015) concur with these findings in their longitudinal study which aimed to explore whether sexual abuse in childhood, between birth and 17.5 years, predicts IPV in adulthood. They discovered that IPV was significantly predicted by abuse in childhood and dissociation arising from CSA (Zamir & Lavee, 2015).

The quality of day-to-day life can also be influenced by one's coping with CSA throughout life. Astbury, Bruck and Loxton (2011), for example, researched the prevalence of sexual abuse and its contribution to sleeping difficulties among Australian women aged 24–30 years. The study was part of the Australian Longitudinal Study on Women's Health involving three age cohorts: young, 18–23 years; middle-aged, 45–50 years; and 70–75 years. The finding was that the higher level of recurrent sleep difficulties experienced by women who report a history of sexual abuse, compared to their non-abused peers, might explain the significant relationship found between forced sex and a range of mental health conditions such as depression, anxiety, self-harm and socio-economic issues such as worries about meeting their financial needs (Astbury et al., 2011).

Easton et al. (2011), in their study of disclosure of sexual abuse by women survivors, discovered that disclosure is rare, and, if they are not believed, there are many and varied negative impacts on subsequent relationships and psychosexual functioning throughout life. The authors telephoned and surveyed research participants who responded to an advertisement distributed through the Centres for Sexual Assault (CASA) in greater Victoria, Australia. The sample consisted of 165 adults (mainly women) who identified as having been sexually abused when they were children. The main aim of the study was to understand the relationship with sexual dysfunction in three main areas: emotional (which included fears of sex, guilt and anxiety about sex); behavioural (touching and arousal); and physical (experiencing satisfaction with sex). Alongside these dimensions, which have been established as important for adult CSA survivors, the authors assessed the relevance of a range of variables including: age at which the sexual abuse occurred, frequency of abuse and duration, relationship between abuser and child, and whether the participant disclosed to anyone about the abuse and the nature of the response from the caregiver. The authors discovered connections with previous research that highlighted the relationship between sexual functioning and the number of sexual abusers, the age at which the abuse occurred and the relationship with the abuser. The conclusion, aligning with past studies, found that the severity of the impact related to the type of sexual contact, the frequency of abuse and the emotional stress due to traumatic sexualisation, particularly if the child or adolescent had an awareness of what was happening. The closer the relationship with the abuser, the younger the age at which the abuse first occurred, the longer the duration of the abuse and the higher the number of occurrences are all factors linked to a higher level of traumatic sexualisation. The presence of these factors working together increases the survivor's sense of powerlessness and the severity of the impact.

The authors conclude:

> Because children expect family members to support and protect them, children who are abused by family members, especially parents, may experience higher levels of traumatic sexualisation and betrayal than children who are sexually abused by non-family members. The heightened sense of betrayal may make it more difficult for children to form healthy intimate relationships during adulthood, contributing to poorer psychosexual functioning.
>
> (Easton et al., 2011, p. 43)

The authors further hypothesised that disclosure of the abuse to a trusted adult might mitigate the severity of the impact of the abuse in terms of psychosexual functioning in adult survivors (Easton et al., 2011, p. 43). The emotional dimensions included fear of sex and guilt during sex; the behavioural dimensions included problems with sexual touching and becoming aroused; the evaluative dimensions related to satisfaction with sexual experience. The results of the study were that only 10 of the 165 participants disclosed the abuse within one week of the abuse, and for most it was more than ten years before the issue was disclosed. Overall, telling another about the abuse had a negative impact on feelings of guilt during sex in adulthood unlike the case for those who did not tell someone. The respondents who were older at the time of their first experience of sexual abuse were more likely to experience problems related to the emotional dimension of sexual functioning than those who were younger at the time of the first abuse. Among those who disclosed about their abuse, this group were approximately eight times more likely to have a problem with sexually touching as adults when they were older at the time of their abuse.

The authors conclude that older children who are abused and disclose may receive a more negative response to their disclosure that may involve being disbelieved by a trusted caregiver, or they may be blamed. Unsupportive responses to disclosure or blaming responses may increase the child or adolescent survivors' feelings of fear, guilt and betrayal that remain with them into their adult life. The type of abuse and relationship with the perpetrator were found to be issues for adult sexual functioning. Incest increased the likelihood of having difficulties with physical touching during adulthood. The authors hypothesise that the attachment to the perpetrator in a parental relationship when connected with acts of sexual abuse increases the likelihood of feelings of betrayal, apprehension and confusion in one's adult sexual functioning (p. 49).

The multivariate model developed by Easton et al. (2011) found that age, severity (in terms of being physically as well as sexually abused/being abused by more than one perpetrator) and telling others about the abuse were important factors in influencing psychosexual functioning in adulthood.

The authors recommend that awareness should be raised of the importance of the response to disclosure, it being important for survivors' future psychosexual functioning and well-being overall to have a supportive response from the helping practitioner. To summarise these research findings, a valuable part of the clinical assessment needs to address the questions in the box to determine the likely impact of any delays in disclosure and to document the potential negative impact of judgements from those trusted adults who were told.

1. What were the duration and frequency of the CSA?
2. What was the nature of the relationship of the survivor to the perpetrator (i.e., was incest involved, which raises a particular risk factor of poor outcomes in adulthood for psychosexual functioning)?
3. How old was the client when the abuse first occurred?
4. How severe was the abuse in terms of duration, frequency and kind of abuse, and did multiple forms of maltreatment and/or CSA feature? (Whether physical abuse or injury, neglect or emotional, psychological, financial or spiritual abuse existed in addition to the sexual abuse alerts practitioners to the likelihood of compounding effects of different forms of abuse which are interlocking.)

A life trajectory perspective

From a perspective of narrative theory, these questions may be reframed by asking what has brought the woman survivor to seek help such as counselling or other forms of therapy. From this major storyline of the current challenge within the life stage or trajectory, the subplot of the sexual abuse may arise. If a history of CSA is offered by the woman, then it is important that this is heard as it is now a part of her major storyline in the telling or retelling to another. How the abuse legacy relates to the current life challenge can then be explored in greater detail. The decision to seek help can be reframed as a choice point to recall the abuse or not to recall it again. Alternatively, the woman survivor may prefer, as Gasker's (1999) women clients did, simply to state she was abused at some point in her childhood and to move on to the present dilemma. This choice point can be discussed from the woman's positioning of being the author of her life, so retaining control of where she wishes to begin her story and the direction in which she wishes to take the storyline in counselling. If the therapist can see a connection of CSA to her personal biography, then these parallels can be offered for further reflection at some point when the therapeutic relationship is sufficiently established and there is sufficient skill in building scaffolding to hear about patterns.

Integrating the past with the present

As illustrated in the previous chapter, some recollections of CSA, when formed too early in the development of the relationship with the helping professional, can have adverse effects. As illustrated in the case of Fiona, a first disclosure in a therapeutic relationship that has not been adequately established can precipitate a flight into avoidance and/or a physical flight from the therapeutic context. While classical Freudian psychoanalysis might term this evidence of a psychological defence, the New Trauma Therapy conceptualises this as a response of returning to strategies involved in childhood coping mechanisms, which themselves need to be respected and honoured (Briere, 1996).

As well as emotional congruence and connection with a trusted other, the physical context and safety are discussed in women survivor accounts of what constitutes safety (Harms, 2015; Gasker, 1999). This suggests that helping professionals need to pay attention to the physical context in which they offer their services. Having a tranquil office setting that is heated adequately and is free from air conditioning and other noise and from distracting odours is, therefore, also important.

Integration refers in narrative terms to a process of incorporating experience into the overall life narrative (Gasker, 1999, p. 38). Following disclosure and exploration of the manifold ways in which the event has impacted the survivor's life, the therapeutic task is to encourage the woman to reframe her experience of what happened so that it is consistent with her identity and the hopes that she holds for her life in the present.

The following case study of Lisa demonstrates a current major life theme – a desire to start a family – followed by the loss of a much-longed-for pregnancy. These traumatic life events evoked themes of earlier child sexual abuse that again became prominent and queued for attention. In the safety of a caring therapeutic relationship, the recent loss prompted a retelling of CSA.

Case study: Lisa

I embarked on my work with Lisa when she was referred by the team at the regional hospital where I work as head of grief and loss counselling. I was asked to see Lisa as a late first-time mother with complications in her current pregnancy at 22 weeks' gestation. The background notes indicated that the medical specialists had established an abnormality in the current pregnancy, and, following genetic counselling, the couple were advised of the diagnosis and the options for continuing or terminating the current pregnancy. Owing to the shock and trauma of the news, a referral to the counselling team, was made.

Lisa is a 41-year-old Asian woman who is happily married to her Pakeha (New Zealander of European descent) husband (John). Both were struggling to come to terms with news of an abnormal pregnancy following a diagnosis of Edwards syndrome, a genetic condition indicating a chromosomal abnormality that is considered to be incompatible with life. The couple had been advised that such a condition rarely results in a live baby following birth and they had been offered the option of terminating the pregnancy. The pregnancy had been conceived naturally after IVF (in vitro fertilisation) had been unsuccessful after one round of treatment. Lisa and John had been referred to a private fertility clinic for treatment when they wished to start a family and realised they were having difficulty conceiving. As the procedures for IVF were invasive, Lisa had decided she could not endure further rounds of fertility treatment.

The difficulties in conceiving a pregnancy had been ongoing for three years after Lisa and John first began trying to have a family. Lisa had met her husband, John, as a 37 year old when he was 55, and the age gap meant that they had decided to try for a family as soon as they knew that this was what they both wanted.

Decision making over the pregnancy

The immediate therapeutic task at hand with Lisa and John was to enable them to work through their shock and feelings of being traumatised at the news of the diagnosis. Moving forward, in the next few weeks, they needed to make a decision about whether to continue or to end the pregnancy through an early induction of labour. A private suite within the hospital was tentatively booked in case the couple wished to take this option. Over three sessions with the couple, I gained a rapport quickly to forge a purposeful relationship with the couple in order to support them in their difficult decision making; they decided that if, on subsequent testing, the diagnosis of Edwards syndrome was confirmed, they would seek the induction of labour. Both were clear that, had the pregnancy been diagnosed as having Trisomy 21, or Downs syndrome, they would have chosen to continue the pregnancy to term and would have raised their child. Upon more sophisticated genetic testing, the diagnosis of Edwards syndrome was confirmed, and so the induction of labour was scheduled and was successfully completed without complication.

I saw Lisa and her husband after the procedure when Lisa had recovered and been discharged from hospital. They were sad but philosophical about their decision and, in retrospect, considered it to be the right decision for them. Lisa said that it was helpful to their grieving process to spend time with their baby, albeit briefly, whom they had named Iris after Lisa's favourite flower that was in bloom in their garden. Iris had had foot and hand castings taken by the nursing staff to be framed for the nursery they had made ready for their baby. This room was now transformed into Lisa's office. John had not wanted to see the baby and had since returned to work. Lisa had taken another three weeks away from her busy professional life as she did not feel ready to reintegrate into the workaday world after such an impactful experience. She described her emotions as still understandably 'raw' and, as a manager, she did not wish to tell colleagues why she had been away on sick leave. Fortunately, no one in her workplace knew of the pregnancy, and so she did not have to explain any details when she returned to work. Being a very private person, having to explain the reasons for her absence would have been very burdensome for her. Lisa found herself avoiding physical affection from her husband as she construed this as an invitation to become sexual and she said lately she 'had not been in the mood'. They had decided to have some couple therapy to come to some decisions about future directions in their lives and explore the impact of the loss of pregnancy.

The epiphany experience for Lisa

During her time off work grieving for the loss of baby Iris, and with couple sessions underway, Lisa told me in my follow-up appointments with her that she had been reflecting upon her life and the impact of incidents of sexual abuse that occurred to her as a ten year old. She advised that she was not sleeping well and was using some sleeping medication prescribed after the loss of her baby. She wanted to talk about a 'light bulb' moment she had had recently. This insight was about the importance of Iris giving her the opportunity to be a different kind of mother in contrast to the experiences of detachment Lisa recalled with her mother as she was growing up.

As Lisa's mother seemed emotionally remote from her as she was growing up, and her father was an inconsistent figure on whom she could not rely, as a ten year old she had developed a relationship with one of his friends who was a fatherlike figure to her. She had been a victim of sexual abuse perpetrated by this family friend, who was at the house repeatedly over a two-year period until they migrated to New Zealand to live. The current trauma of the loss of pregnancy and the hope for a baby seemed to have led to an epiphany where the powerlessness of the current experience evoked memories from the past. Lisa said it was this feeling of powerlessness that was throwing her life into crisis. On the day she disclosed this connection to me, her car had broken down on the way to the hospital unexpectedly, and she was almost an hour late for her appointment. The receptionist found her weeping in the waiting room and so brought her down to my office owing to her distress. Between sobs she said that, 'even the car lets me down'.

She had told her mother, in recent weeks, about her experiences of childhood sexual abuse. Lisa's mother, who is a devout Buddhist, tried to philosophise the experience away, to say that these things happen for a reason, and that these kinds of experiences, while difficult, once navigated, make a person stronger. For Lisa, she felt anger again for not being heard or validated. During the induced labour in hospital, Lisa had her mother on Skype to offer support, though, once again, she had felt her mother was distant, reassuring her that the loss of pregnancy was 'for the best' rather than hearing Lisa's despair about the diagnosis and the impossible decision she and her husband had had to make.

The therapeutic goal of disclosure with validation

Following the guidance of recent theorists drawn on throughout this chapter, I noted that Lisa was attempting to integrate her past abuse experiences with the current life events of relationship commitment, decision to start a family, pregnancy and loss of pregnancy. Lisa's realisation about the impact of CSA in the context of these life stage events came as a moment of insight. This realisation was a gradual dawning in the context of grief after losing her daughter, highlighting her earlier relationship with her mother and the experience of being disbelieved as a child. In grieving for the loss of her baby Iris, when her husband had moved on in his grief by returning to work, she had an epiphany experience of recalling not being validated by her mother during the recent time of diagnosis of the genetic abnormality of her pregnancy. The traumatic decision to end the pregnancy and the loss of the pregnancy were told to her mother, who minimised her experience. This minimising response mirrored being disbelieved about her child sexual abuse as a ten year old. Following those recent experiences of invalidation by her mother, Lisa searched for validation of the recent events and those from her childhood past. A choice point to retell her abuse narrative came when she was re-traumatised by her mother's lack of empathy. This lack of acknowledgement had compounded her sense of powerlessness in the current situation of finding the pregnancy was abnormal and making the impossible decision of ending her much-longed-for first pregnancy with her husband.

Her grief was compounded by the fact that she felt she had left pregnancy until 'too late'. She felt that her life goal of starting a family with her husband was no longer relevant, and that their life needed to be heading in a new direction. She told me that they had decided not to try for another pregnancy. They were planning to take time out of their careers to travel and to live overseas for a few years and would let their home to tenants to finance their adventure. Lisa was looking forward to visiting countries they had not been to before. Lisa said she was applying for jobs overseas. Lisa and John were looking forward to reconnecting with people they knew overseas, including her mother, who had shifted back to care for elderly parents. Lisa's new life direction was an attempt at re-authoring when the former life no longer seemed relevant.

Conclusion: integration of present with past life themes

The process of integration of a positive self-image in which one has authorship of one's life and some semblance of control over one's life is one of the major therapeutic tasks. In the case study of Lisa and her history of CSA, the current life stage and decision to have children emphasised Lisa's wish to transcend her personal narrative as a survivor of CSA and become a different mother figure to her child when she had reflected on her experiences with her own mother. This wish to become a better parent when there is a history of CSA is a common legacy of CSA, particularly when there is a lack of protection and intervention by the non-offending parent or guardian. Being disbelieved by the non-offending parent when disclosing CSA hampers further attempts to tell, which can mean that the abuse continues without this protection and intervention to stop the CSA.

In summary, connections with previous research have highlighted the relationship between adult functioning and the age at which abuse was experienced and the relationship with the abuser as predicting the aftermath of abuse in adulthood. The conclusion that the severity of the impact is related to the type of sexual contact and frequency means, therefore, that it is important that practitioners assess these. The emotional stress due to traumatic sexualisation, particularly if the child or adolescent had an awareness of what was happening, is another theme to be enquired about by clinicians. The closer the relationship with the abuser and the age at first abuse of a longer duration and frequency have been linked to a higher level of traumatic impact as adults (Easton et al., 2011).

For Lisa, the liminal space in which she came to grief and loss counselling after a loss of pregnancy was a place for revisiting past disclosure of CSA as a way of viewing the old life without the new direction being known. We discussed her current life goals and being at the crossroads of change without knowing what the change would be, and, within this pause for reflection, there presented an opportunity to revisit an invalidated response to a first telling of CSA to her mother. In the retelling, she again remembered feeling minimised and realised her life needed to change with the goal of motherhood less relevant to her now. The importance of her relationship with her husband

and a reformulated vision for the future now fuelled her rebounding from the pregnancy loss. As in Cath Bennett's account of abuse as a teen (2018), Lisa was tackling her mother's and society's disbelief about CSA, which she no longer saw as being her fault but saw as an abuse of power by a trusted adult to whom she looked for support as a child.

In the next chapter, we look at the nature of attachment, which is an important variable in the survivor's decision to tell and retell their narrative of CSA.

References

Astbury, J., Bruck, D., & Loxton, D. (2011). Forced sex: a critical factor in the sleep difficulties of young Australian women. *Violence and Victims*, 26(1), 53–72. doi:10.1891/0886-6708.26.1.53

Becker, K. D., Stuewig, J., & McCloskey, L. A. (2010). Traumatic stress symptoms of women exposed to different forms of childhood victimization and intimate partner violence. *Journal of Interpersonal Violence* 25(9), 1699–1715.

Bennett, C. (2018). Moment of reckoning. *Next Magazine*, December, 37–41.

Brazelton, J. F. (2015a). African American women looking back: making meaning of the disclosure process of incest survivors across the life course. (AAI3432702). Retrieved from http://search.proquest.com/docview/1018338865?accountid=14782

Brazelton, J. F. (2015b). The secret storm: exploring the disclosure process of African American women survivors of child sexual abuse across the life course. *Traumatology*, 21(3), 181–187. doi:10.1037/trm0000047

Briere, J. (1996). *Therapy for Adults Molested as Children: Beyond Survival* (2nd ed., revised and expanded). New York: Springer.

Courtois, C. A. (1997). Healing the incest wound: a treatment update with attention to recovered-memory issues. *American Journal of Psychotherapy*, 51(4), 464–496.

Dalenberg, C. (2000). *Countertransference and the Treatment of Trauma*. La Jolla, CA: American Psychological Association.

Easton, S. D., Coohey, C., O'Leary, P., Zhang, Y., & Hua, L. (2011). The effect of childhood sexual abuse on psychosexual functioning during adulthood. *Journal of Family Violence*, 26, 41–50. doi:10.1007/s10896-010-9340-6

Epston, D., & White, M. (1992). *Experience, Contradiction, Narrative and Imagination: Selected Papers of David Epston and Michael White, 1989–1991*. Adelaide: Dulwich Centre.

Gasker, J. A. (1999). *I Never Told Anyone This Before: Managing the Initial Disclosure of Sexual Abuse Re-collections*. Routledge.

Geertz, C. (1975). *The Interpretation of Cultures: Selected Essays*. Basic Books.

Gitterman, C., & Germain, A. (2008). *The Life Model of Social Work Practice: Advances in Theory and Practice* (3rd ed.). New York: Colombia University Press.

Harms, L. (2015). *Understanding Trauma and Resilience*. London: Palgrave Macmillan.

Herman, J. L. (1992). *Trauma and Recovery*. New York: Basic Books.

Leibrich, J. (2015). *Sanctuary: The Discovery of Wonder*. Dunedin: Otago University Press.

Mooney, J. L., & McGregor, C. (2018). How adults tell: messages for society and policy makers regarding disclosures of childhood sexual abuse. Unpublished PhD thesis. School of Political Science and Sociology, National University of Ireland, Galway.

Myerhoff, B. G. (1982). *Number Our Days: Triumph of Continuity and Culture among Jewish Old People in an Urban Ghetto.* New York: Simon & Schuster/Touchstone Books.

Pearlman, L. A., & Saakvitne, K. W. (1995). *Trauma and the Therapist: Countertransference and Vicarious Traumatization in Psychotherapy with Incest Survivors.* W.W. Norton.

Salzberg, S. (2017). *Real Love. The Art of Mindful Connection.* New York: Flatiron Books.

Van der Kolk, B. A., McFarlane, A. C., & Weisaeth, L. (Eds.). (1996). *Traumatic Stress: The Effects of Overwhelming Experience on Mind, Body, and Society.* Guilford Press.

White, M., (1995). *Re-Authoring Lives: Interviews and Essays.* Adelaide: Dulwich Centre.

White, M., & Epston, D. (1990). *Narrative Means to Therapeutic Ends.* New York: W. W. Norton.

Zamir, O., & Lavee, Y. (2015). Emotional awareness and breaking the cycle of revictimization. *Journal of Family Violence*, 30, 675–684.

3 The role of relationship in women's disclosure of CSA

> I had a strong reaction to hearing her disclose what happened, a very strong reaction. It came after working for it for years, but it came in writing. She couldn't verbalise it in words yet. We both knew there was a lot there to be elicited but she was very, very, very dissociated and a lot of her therapy has been done in writing and there's a part of her that is able to write it very eloquently, with enormous impact. [Pause to reflect] Mmm. Yes. Very powerful material, that was huge for me to hear and read and take in.
>
> (Pack, 2002, 175–176)

A trauma counsellor, Beth, discusses a first disclosure from a 35-year-old woman client who had a long history of CSA but could not verbalise her abuse safely owing to dissociating while remembering. She started writing about her abuse and its impact after many years of therapeutic work together with Beth as her therapist.

Introduction

The above was recounted to me in the course of earlier research with sexual abuse therapists about the most difficult issue brought to them by their clients who were survivors of CSA (Pack, 2002). For Beth, it was knowing that her client, Marnie, wished to discuss details of her abuse with her but could not yet verbalise this. Owing to the level of dissociation Marnie experienced when thinking about the abuse (which was father–daughter incest), recollections of her abuse were unavailable as a coherent narrative. Beth realised that the therapeutic work needed to be carefully paced so that Marnie was not re-traumatised by the remembering process or by disclosing too soon for her. Recollecting and disclosing too soon can prompt re-traumatisation where past memories of abuse are re-experienced in the present. Marnie had never been able to disclose to anyone any details of what had happened with her father owing to shame and dissociation. Father–daughter incest is considered to be one of the most sensitive for counsellors to grapple with according to the New Trauma therapists of the previous chapters (Briere, 1996; Herman, 1992). Intuiting this, Beth, guided by the trauma-informed theory of the New

DOI: 10.4324/9781032669205-3

Trauma therapists, suggested a writing methodology to help in the planning for disclosure of CSA in a way that she thought might feel somewhat safer to Marnie than an impromptu verbal disclosure. Marnie was a successful policy writer for a government department, and so Beth's encouraging her to journal between sessions and bring her journal to each session to review capitalised on Marnie's skills and abilities in this therapeutic methodology. With the week-by-week meeting to review the writing and the writing process, this structure formed a solid platform for Marnie's processing of what came up week by week in terms of feelings and thoughts about her recollections. What happened between sessions was informative of the relationship between client and therapist, as Marnie told Beth that she felt the supportive presence of Beth standing alongside her as she recalled and wrote.

Beth's comments above highlight the way in which the relationship with women survivors of CSA can provide a safe container within which client and therapist together find a way of making the unspeakable speakable or, in this case, writeable. The ways in which connection allows for historical disclosure of CSA, as well as exploration of the process that happens after disclosure is made, are the focus of this chapter. Dissociation, common to many adults traumatised as children and adolescents by CSA, is thought to rob survivors of their verbal capacities as their abuse triggers a splitting of the mind and body to cope, making memory fragmented and not experienced as a coherent whole. The process of writing things down and bringing them to therapy week by week enabled Marnie to express herself in a way that felt safe. This relationship found a creative means of facilitating the telling and retelling of the narrative of her relationship with family members within which her CSA occurred over many years of her childhood. This process of remembering permits other versions of self and other to be explored in a non-judgemental way. Though the incest with her father had never been formally reported to the authorities, or anyone else when she was an adult, the possibility of reconnection with her father had triggered a life crisis where the ambivalence of the relationship with him was rekindled, awaiting attention in the hope of a resolution to enable Marnie to move on with her life.

The supportive, allowing attitude of Beth as her counsellor removed the imperative to do or say anything, which in itself may be enough to transform the emotional and psychological pain of the legacy of childhood sexual abuse. The hallmarks of CSA are usually coercion and the misuse of adult power over the child who was looking to the parent or primary attachment figure for consistency of care, including emotional congruence and responsiveness to the needs of the child. As Beth had established a relationship through empathetic engagement, she had suggested the process of writing recollections and reflections. In so doing, Beth had established a methodology with her client in a co-created partnership. Disclosure of what happened in Marnie's childhood took many years, and, through going at the client's pace, they reached a milestone in the healing journey through writing and reading of writing, week by week, in therapy. The planning for disclosure was important throughout this process, as was the therapeutic relationship, with Beth guiding the pacing of the disclosure process collaboratively with Marnie. Any hierarchical or top–down approach in which Marnie felt her voice was not heard would have made disclosure impossible as, during feelings of powerlessness, Beth observed that Marnie withdrew into herself and became watchful and silent. The prospect of seeing her father after many years of absence meant that Marnie wanted to explore her feelings towards him, which involved her abuse memories and grief at the loss of innocence in childhood.

A relational approach to disclosure

Having the safety of a trusting relationship to facilitate disclosure of historical abuse for adult women who are survivors of CSA is essential to the process of remembering. In some instances, an inpatient setting that provides a team of supportive professionals may take the place of a single therapeutic relationship. It may be an entire team that provides the safe haven in which to disclose. The inpatient experience also takes the survivor out of the day-to-day setting of her everyday life. This may be beneficial in providing neutral ground away from memories and associations of the places where the original abuse occurred and the significant others who were involved. The facilitator of safety for disclosure to occur is the relationship the woman has with the person disclosed to. This relationship can provide the 'secure base' (Winnicott, 1965) from which the disclosure narrative can be told. It is the nature and quality of this relationship that we will now move on to explore.

Knowledge of attachment styles and early family functioning

Attachment theory is at the base of our understanding as to why someone feels safe enough to disclose to another. Winnicott, a British paediatrician and psychoanalyst, in his now classic work of the 'good enough' mother, theorised that a stable caregiver provides the developing infant with the consistent relationship that is needed to internalise an understanding of others in adulthood (Winnicott, 1965). Through experimenting with new situations, the child is using the internalised role of this relationship in order to take the role of the other (Winnicott, 1965). This primary caregiver relationship enables trust and a belief in the other and in broader relationships in the world. This concept of the 'good enough mother' has been extended in subsequent theorising from the traditional mother figure to the emotionally appropriate and responsive caregiver, who may be an extended family member, peer, friend, teacher or significant other to the child (Wallis & Woodworth, 2021). In terms of disclosure, a relationship with a trusted other provides the safe space in which to reflect about past abuse and to troubleshoot the way forward.

An understanding of how attachment styles develop in childhood provides practitioners with a framework for knowing how to build a relationship when there are anxieties variously expressed by women survivors of CSA about being let down, abandoned and/or disbelieved in the therapeutic relationship. Increasingly, as the stigma of discussing one's sexual abuse is challenged by lobby groups and advocates, as in the #MeToo movement, more women than ever before may feel entitled to seek some form of professional help to discuss historical CSA. Therefore, in dealing with disclosures of CSA from adult survivors, it is helpful for practitioners to have an understanding of the different attachment styles as this knowledge base can assist in developing and maintaining the therapeutic relationship, in expectation that these anxieties are likely to colour and emerge as a theme at any stage in their contact with women survivors.

The term 'secure base' refers to the child's need for an early affectional bond between the child and their caregiver. Ideally, the child is responded to in a way that is consistent and emotionally congruent. Through this 'secure base', a child is able to moderate their fears and emotions associated with exploration and new situations, seeking reassurance and comfort from a consistent caregiver. Bowlby's theory of childhood attachment assumes that the secure base is internalised through 'internal working models' (Bowlby, 1973). The biological parent, step-parent or parental figure in a child's life develops affectional ties with the child through such bonds. Bowlby further hypothesised that this pattern of interaction between adult parent and child develops into a 'caregiving bond' (Howe, 2011, p. 11, summarising the work of Bowlby and Winnicott). Early theorists such as Bowlby (1973) and Winnicott (1965) saw this relationship between the primary parent/caregiver and child as representing both a refuge, within which the child can experiment with behaviour through a dynamic interaction with the parent, and the 'secure base' from which to learn to develop emotionally (Howe, 2011, pp. 18–19). Where this 'secure base' is not established, the child can develop anxiety about being alone in the world, hampering the development of an internal working model that guides behaviour through an internalised sense of what to do and how to react in any given context and situation. An understanding of the various styles of attachment develops out of one's internalised working model established during childhood. This internal working model continues to be mirrored in adult relationships with friends, partners, children and extended family.

Attachment styles

The five types of attachment styles classically described by Mary Ainsworth, who was an associate and colleague of Bowlby, involve the classification system developed following her experimental observational studies of a mother and her child. In these studies, a mother was asked to engage in playing with her child and then was asked to leave the room. The departure of the mother and the cessation of her interaction in play prompted a challenge for her child as they suddenly find themself alone in a strange environment. The mother of the child was asked to enter the room after a period of time to reconnect with her child. The behaviour of the child on being left alone and then greeted again by the mother was then recorded by the team.

The various responses of the child to the differing scenarios of being left alone and being engaged with by the mother were found to be representative of one of the five types of attachment. During Ainsworth's research, she discovered that children displayed behaviours associated with the styles shown in the box.

Five styles of attachment

1. Secure attachment (Type B): this style of attachment is described by the scenario where the child in Ainsworth's experiment responds initially with high levels of eye contact and interaction with the mother when played with. The child cries when the mother is asked to leave the room and is observed to be soothed in the presence of the mother when she returns to the room. The care given by the mother is deemed in this scenario to be sensitive to the child's emotional needs, and the mother is seen as being responsive in a consistent and appropriate way with her child. The child is more engaged and actively seeks the interaction of the mother over that of the teaching assistant who was asked to enter the room to interact with the child.
2. Insecure or avoidant attachment (Type A): in this scenario, the child does not demonstrate any sign of distress when the mother departs from the room. There is no strong preference for the mother over a research assistant, and the child avoids or ignores the mother when she re-enters the room. The child remains watchful and disengaged in the presence of the mother.
3. Insecure and ambivalent attachment (Type C): in this scenario, the child becomes very distressed when the mother leaves the room and continues to be inconsolable when she returns. The child runs towards the parent when she leaves but may angrily reject attempts to connect to console and soothe when the mother approaches to pacify the child's angst.
4. Insecure and disorganised attachment (Type D): in this scenario, the child remains both ambivalent and avoidant towards the mother upon re-entry to the room. The child tends to see the mother as being unavailable as a source of support to them and may show signs that they are frightened of her by freezing in her presence as they are conflicted about the emotional availability and responsiveness of their mother towards them.
5. Non-attachment: in this scenario, the child shows no sign of any attachment. This attachment style is typically associated with those children who are raised in institutional care where there has not been any opportunity for interaction with a caregiver. The child looks to the mother for basic needs to be met but does not see the availability of emotional interaction or support.

(Summary of Ainsworth's attachment categories; Howe, 2011, pp. 79–80)

With the styles of attachment outlined, we will look at how these styles manifest in the case study of Stella at the end of this chapter. Suffice it to say here that women who have had their disclosures of CSA rejected, disbelieved or minimised by their mother or primary caregiver may typically withdraw and avoid and so, in their adult behaviour, they may demonstrate some features of the Type A attachment style. Alternatively they may demonstrate insecure and ambivalent attachment styles towards caregivers within the family owing to the disbelief and/or lack of response from significant others (Type C). This ambivalence then enters the therapeutic relationship and is enacted with the professional helper.

In situations where there is ongoing abuse by parental figures over many years, there may be functioning in adulthood based on more insecure, ambivalent and disorganised styles (Type D). It may be difficult to engage with women operating in the Type D style as, typically, they may need to focus on skill building for emotional regulation prior to engaging in abuse recovery work.

This is not to suggest that women survivors of CSA may have just one style established in childhood, as there are multiple trajectories across the life course where the buffering protective factors in the woman's adult life may mean the earlier internal working model is adapted and worked from. Some survivors may demonstrate and work from all the styles, depending on the stage in the therapeutic rapport building or context. Therefore, the attachment styles may be more malleable and fluid than the typology of styles suggests. The attachment styles are not mutually exclusive, and, depending on context, one or more styles may be demonstrated in a particular stage or trajectory of life, depending on what current challenge is arising in the life narrative.

Differing cultural definitions of 'family'

With the cautions above about the limitations of any model and its ability to describe complex human behaviour, so, too, is it necessary to redefine earlier understandings of terms such as 'family'. The notions of 'family' and 'caregiver' may have different definitions across cultures, beyond the nuclear family of parents and their offspring. For example, within Māoridom in Aotearoa New Zealand, attachment may be understood within the contexts mentioned above and include broader relationships within *whānau* (extended family), *hāpu* (or subtribe) and *iwi* (related to one's wider tribal affiliations). Similarly, Pacific cultures have broader understandings of family and parenting, where a child may be given to an extended family member to be raised as a normal part of family life. The social workers who are registered to practice in Aotearoa New Zealand are expected to have competencies in working biculturally and to advocate for Māori as part of their professional registration (Social Workers Registration Board, 2013).

An understanding of the colonial past impacting extended family relationships is, therefore, needed when working with family disclosures and for these cultural definitions, overlaying the attachment theory with culturally relevant understandings of such terms as 'parent' and 'family'. It is important that practitioners become more knowledgeable about research that seeks to explore the impact of colonisation on many First Nations people. Professionals also need a background understanding of the original treaties and agreements between colonial governments and the indigenous people of the land if they are lacking a lived experience of being colonised. How intergenerational trauma can be a feature for CSA survivors who are *tangāta whenua*, or the indigenous 'people of the land', introduces a broader context within which a history of CSA may be set (Pack, 2009). These themes will be discussed in the case study of Stella and in the conclusion at the end of this chapter.

With an understanding of attachment and attachment styles, we now move on to current thinking about attachment and its role in disclosure of CSA for adult women. Themes include attachment and attachment styles delaying or facilitating disclosure, the availability of the non-offending caregiver as a moderating or protective factor in disclosure of CSA and the family dynamics as hampering or facilitating disclosure.

Applications of attachment theory to understanding the disclosure of CSA

The classic theorising about attachment has more recently been applied to the disclosure of CSA. The themes of this literature include: the need to identify attachment styles developed in childhood, the availability of the 'secure base' and assessing the balance of risk and protective factors in the woman's past and current life. For example, Karakurt and Silver (2014) recommend reference to attachment theory when assisting women survivors of childhood sexual abuse. An attachment framework grounded in the foundational work of Bowlby (1973), they argue, assists in identifying attachment styles that have developed in childhood. Reference to the attachment styles summarised above has the potential to explain the reasons why children develop different patterns of interaction with caregivers dependent on the varying availability of a 'secure base'. These internalised 'working models' enable a stable sense of self by which the child can interpret and predict experiences in adult relationships, and these working models are likely to impact the therapeutic relationship in the present when working with adult survivors (Karakurt & Silver, 2014, p. 81). Subsequent researchers on Bowlby's theories of attachment have discovered that the presence of any consistent caregiver figure can act to buffer the more negative impacts of CSA for adult survivors (Godbout et al, 2014). This finding suggests an expansion of the 'good enough mother' to the 'good enough' responsible adult relationship, more broadly.

Karakurt and Silver (2014) also recommend a systemic family focus as being important to the healing of women from the legacy of CSA. Ecological systems theory, from which many models of family therapy derive, focuses on the parts of the system and how they operate together to influence the environment in which the family lives. The ways that family members communicate are indicative of the patterns of interaction that can problematize some members of the family or some of their behaviours. We will explore the family systems approach more fully in forthcoming chapters in relation to narrative approaches and narrative theory. Suffice it to say here that these dynamics of the original family system can operate to support the perpetrator and, in so doing, silence the victim of the abuse from speaking about the abuse, leading to the historical disclosure of CSA (Karakurt & Silver, 2014).

Wallis and Woodworth (2021) discovered in their research that individuals with avoidant styles of attachment in childhood and lack of caregiver engagement significantly delayed disclosure. Extensive abuse over time also acted to delay disclosure, with the support of non-abusing caregivers found to be a mitigating factor. If there was a supportive caregiver within the family in relation to the survivor, this relationship was deemed to have a protective effect on the child with regard to disclosure. The authors conclude that parental reactions are central to whether a child will make a disclosure of their abuse or delay disclosure. The support of caregivers or parental-type figures as alternatives to parents, if the parents are unavailable, is considered central to the understanding of why some children disclose and why disclosures of CSA are delayed until a later time in life. Important in the decision to disclose is the child's assessment of the availability of emotional support in the aftermath of disclosure, which has hitherto been a neglected area of the CSA disclosure literature (Wallis & Woodworth, 2021). Direct questioning by a trusted caregiver was the recommended way of eliciting disclosure from children and to avoid delayed disclosure in adulthood. If disclosure is significantly delayed, their participants found that this often means evidence is lost with the passage of time, which leads to a lack of success with formal disclosure to the authorities and, ultimately, a loss of legal redress (Wallis & Woodworth, 2021).

Attachment styles and CSA

Recent research has identified different factors in the original family functioning that can provide the context for different attachment styles impacting the disclosure of CSA. These attachment styles were found to affect the woman's mental health subsequently. For example, Canton-Cortes et al. (2015) examined the effects of secure, avoidant and anxious attachment styles on depressive symptomatology in adult women who had historical CSA. A total of 168 women were surveyed using a self-reported questionnaire that incorporated the Beck Depression Inventory to assess depression. The attachment style was assessed using the attachment style measure (ASM). The results were that the variables of type of abuse, the relationship with the perpetrator and whether the abuse was continuous or 'one-off' affected the attachment style. This is an important finding as attachment style can affect every facet of the adult women's life. Parenting, romantic relationships and the durability of peer and partner relationships can be impacted by the aftermath of CSA for women survivors. Canton-Cortes et al.'s analysis of prior studies of attachment and the role of attachment styles for women survivors has found that secure attachment styles can serve to regulate negative affect and act as a protective factor to lower anxiety in the face of stressful life events. Their research confirms that a secure attachment style was related to lower scores on depression among the survivors of CSA. There was no relationship, however, between avoidant attachment style and depression (Canton-Cortes et al., 2015, p. 433) or when the abuse was rated as being more severe, such as ongoing abuse by a parental figure. The role of attachment styles and their impact upon the development of depression for adult survivors of CSA depended on the type of abuse experienced, the duration of the abuse (isolated or continuing) and the relationship to the perpetrator of the abuse. In cases of oral or penetrative sex that had been an isolated event, the effects on attachment style were more evident. The onset of depressive symptoms in adulthood was found to be greater with this kind of sexual abuse. The authors surmise that depressive symptomatology cannot be explained by individual adjustment traits but that the characteristics of the type and severity of abuse may lead to disclosure of CSA in childhood, which is a protective factor in adulthood. In contact with helping professionals, therapeutic strategies that are recommended are those aimed at building secure relationships in which the type, extent and duration of abuse can be assessed safely. Trust in the therapeutic relationship may be more difficult to build where the abuse was oral/penetrative, the abuse had occurred outside the immediate family and it was a single rather than repeated event (Canton-Cortes et al., 2015, p. 433).

The role of relationship in disclosing CSA while in residential treatment facilities

While most women survivors seek historical disclosure in the community at a time of their choosing, with a trusted adult or a health or counselling professional, there are those disclosures that are enabled by a safe residential setting and multidisciplinary team. For example, Miller's research found that, for women with diagnosed eating disorders, 60% disclosed CSA while in residential care when asked by their treating clinicians about childhood sexual abuse (Miller, 1993). The author reports that less than half of the perpetrators were reported to anyone within one year of the occurrence of sexual abuse, and two-thirds of the disclosures had been made to family, peers and friends. Following disclosure as inpatients, women in the residential therapy group researched were reported to have experienced shame or guilt. Some of the reasons given for choosing not to disclose CSA earlier were related to fears that those disclosed to would not understand, believe and/or do anything about the abuse. These fears were strongly felt in relation to parents of the women who were under treatment for bulimia or anorexia nervosa. The author further found that the most serious sexual abuse (in terms of force associated with the abuse, threats and coercion) was reported more to peers/acquaintances than to parents. Furthermore, almost half of disclosures of CSA to parents did result in some negative implications for the survivor. These negative impacts ranged from a lack of empathy to humiliation or lack of intervention to address the abuse (Miller, 1993). Overall, the majority of disclosures to supporters outside the family received positive or neutral responses (Miller, 1993).

These patterns of disclosure are echoed in other studies and so are not unique to women who are being treated for eating disorders. The findings of such studies indicate the clinical importance of enquiring about prior disclosures: why the woman did or did not disclose, what the reaction was from those disclosed to, and perceptions and feelings about others' responses. Twelve per cent of women surveyed for the first time chose to disclose in the residential treatment setting (Miller, 1993). This finding supports those of other researchers whose research suggests that the reasons for disclosure include whether there was direct questioning by counsellors and encouragement by others in the survivors' social networks to explore what happened in their past (Domhardt et al., 2015, p. 489). The therapeutic value of women survivors attending ongoing therapy groups or therapeutic communities in a residential setting is suggested when questions are directly posed to participants about whether CSA was a feature of their childhood. Among the benefits of this residential or longer-term-outpatient approach is that there is a team and a supportive community surrounding the individual woman survivor. This can be particularly helpful when disclosure causes a crisis for the woman or where self-harm and suicidal ideation can feature. A residential environment can provide a safe place in which to disclose where the aftermath of disclosure can be processed in an ongoing way, with the potential for self-harm monitored and the availability of inpatient stays assisting in the wider treatment plan.

Facilitating disclosure by the use of differing questioning styles: the role of the non-offending supporter

Where there is a history of CSA involving physical violence, force, coercion and/or threats to the child survivor, it can be more difficult to provide the secure base from which the adult woman feels confident enough to disclose the background and history of abuse in the distant past. Miller (1993) discovered that, when women were asked about childhood sexual abuse, they often needed more detailed, overlapping questions about what they understood to be sexual abuse. This conversation may have created the context for prompting questions about their feelings about what they had experienced within the disclosed events. This framing of questions allowed forgotten events to safely re-emerge and to be explored alongside the ways in which the survivor had learned to deal with the CSA subsequently. An assessment as to whether the survivor tended to minimise the events during early years in order to get through the experience could be investigated. This kind of enquiry then framed and contextualised a discussion about the various impacts experienced in the years after the original events, during adolescence and adulthood. The researchers and clinicians in Miller's (1993) study found that they needed to define what sexual abuse is in all its possible forms. The descriptions given to participants defining CSA included non-contact sexual abuse, sexual grooming and abuse involving physical contact. These descriptions were given at the outset of the research to see if these definitions triggered an identification by the survivor with particular parts of what was described. Miller (1993) further found that giving rating scales for the survivor to complete on paper meant that some women denied that they had been abused but, when in a relationship with the interviewer, disclosed their abuse which had earlier been minimised or denied (Miller, 1993). This suggests again that enabling a secure base though a relationship that is supportive, trusting and non-judgemental is pivotal to the process of disclosure. Once women in the residential facility disclosed in the course of the research, they were more open to discussing these incidents and their impact in subsequent adulthood in individual or group therapies that were provided in the eating disorders treatment programme (Miller, 1993, p. 49).

Attachment to non-abusing caregivers and their role in enabling disclosure

Wallis and Woodworth (2021), in their study of the role of the non-abusing caregiver(s) and their role in disclosure, illustrate the ways in which the support of an adult in a caregiving role with the child who is being abused can act as a protective factor in facilitating the disclosure of CSA. This non-offending caregiver, when supportive, is considered to be an important resource who can act to mitigate the impact of children and adolescents delaying disclosure for fear they will break up the family home and the relationship between the parents. If this relationship with the non-offending caregiver continues into adolescence and adulthood from childhood, women have a source of support that may be critical to the ongoing CSA healing journey that is continuing. Wallis and Woodworth (2021) found that the supportive behaviours critical to disclosure involve an unwavering belief in what the survivor says and protecting the survivor by appropriate behaviours such as being available as a sounding board, giving advice and unconditional support.

These dimensions of support from childhood can continue to function as a protective relationship involving an ongoing supportive dialogue across the lifespan. Treating practitioners are recommended to assess and work with such support networks where they are available. Therefore, this requires a broader view of family, looking outside the immediate family to extended family, and, in the case of Māori and Pacific clients, the tribal or *iwi*, subtribal or *hāpu* and extended family or *whānau* can be useful sources of such support. Beyond these blood lines, sports coaches, teachers, peers and significant others may prove to be valuable sources of support in the women survivors' healing. Hergass found in her research that preschool educators were the unexpected recipients of disclosure by abused children from deprived backgrounds living in remote Aboriginal communities in Australia. The preschool educators noticed the children's 'big behaviours' and elicited disclosure by asking about their artwork. They had an ongoing influence in the children's lives, as Hergass found they had a role as a surrogate caregiver to the children. Because of cultural taboos, the children's abuse was not disclosed to their families for a variety of reasons. The parents and other family members had experiences of intergenerational trauma as members of the 'stolen generation' (Hergass, 2019).

In the case study below, the role of the extended family and, in particular, an aunt features in the disclosure of CSA. Owing to the extent of her abuse, Stella had ongoing problems in adulthood because of dissociation, self-harm and suicide attempts. A note to readers: there is some material in this case study that might be triggering for those on their own healing journey, and so these readers may wish to skip to the conclusion to avoid any potential for becoming vicariously traumatised in the engagement with this material.

Case study: Stella's story

Stella is a 25-year-old woman born in New Zealand whose parents migrated from Western Samoa in 1976. She was referred to community mental health services with ongoing self-harming behaviours and dissociation after successful treatment for an eating disorder soon after attaining puberty at the age of 14 years. She had had a long history of contact with the mental health services since the age of 16 when she was diagnosed with an eating disorder involving both anorexia and bulimia nervosa. Stella's eating disorder involved the dual behaviours of fasting alternating with a binge-eating and purging cycle. This cycle was punctuated by excessive exercising (walking 20 kilometres at a stretch). During her dissociative episodes, she would find herself cutting her body in an unconscious state. At other times, she was cognisant of what she was doing and was cutting herself in an effort to self-soothe. The eating disorder was no longer the main presenting problem for her. There had been a legacy from her excessive exercising, however, as she had significant joint problems for which she was attending a pain management clinic within the hospital.

When I met Stella, I noticed she had an old scar running horizontally across her throat that was related to a past suicide attempt in her late teens, of which she had no memory. Hospital staff reported the injury as being self-inflicted as she had tried to cut her own throat with a knife. Her psychiatrist, in the notes on file, mentioned that Stella was troubled by dissociation when she was stressed or when she began reliving memories of past abuse. At these times, she experienced acute psychoses and engaged in self-harming behaviours. The range of self-harming behaviours included cutting, overdosing on her antidepressant medication and walking out into the path of oncoming cars. The notes further indicated that she had been discharged from the mental health services as she was no longer engaging in these destructive and self-harming behaviours. She was not considered to be a high suicide risk at present.

In her history, both Stella and her sister, Vaiula, were sexually abused by a stepfather after her mother divorced their birth father. Stella was aged around five years when the sexual abuse first occurred, and it stopped at the age of 11 years when a concerned aunt elicited a disclosure of CSA from Stella, having for some years been suspicious of what was happening with her sister's new live-in partner. Having been investigated by the child protection services, the matter was referred to the police, and the stepfather was convicted and sentenced for numerous offences involving Stella and her younger sister, who was only four at the time of her abuse. As their mother had her own mental health issues, she remained detached emotionally and, owing to her disengagement from her daughters, was unable to protect them. Stella tried to protect her younger sister from being abused by their stepfather by sacrificing her own safety. When Stella tried to tell her mother what was happening, she was disbelieved by her and so internalised the abuse as being her fault. This shame and self-blame allowed the behaviour of the stepfather to continue. The abuse involved incest through to molestation and physical threats and abuse. Furthermore, the abuse involved her stepfather introducing Stella to his male friends where she was used as a sexual object by groups of his friends and gang raped on more than one occasion. Her eating disorder was an attempt to have some semblance of control over her life where little personal agency was possible for Stella and her sister. The two sisters were taken out of their biological mother's care by the child protection services and they were both placed with their aunt for the remainder of their childhood and adolescence. Aunt Violet, as well as being a more emotionally consistent caregiver, worked in the social services and was raising children from her own marriage to her partner and so could provide the girls with a supportive extended family.

Stella had successfully dealt with her eating disorder to the point that she was now of normal body weight; however, she was observed by her psychiatrist to slip into the alters. The term 'alters' refers to denied parts of self or internalised voices of significant others which emerge and are enacted by the survivor as part of a dissociative process. The alters who emerged were that of an older man who wished to punish her, alternating with a five-year-old girl who wanted her mother and cried as she was 'afraid'. She was no longer under any form of therapeutic group or individual contact with the mental health services and was relatively happy with many aspects of her life.

To her credit, and with her aunt Violet's support, Stella had moved out of supported housing into an independent flat and had a boyfriend (Geoffrey) whom she had met while living in hostel accommodation. He also had a history of psychiatric service contact, and so they had some shared experience of early childhood trauma. Both he and Stella worked as caregivers assisting elderly rest-home residents, a job they both greatly appreciated. Geoffrey wanted to move into live with Stella. Stella had her own flat and lived there alone with her two cats. The prospect of an intimate relationship seemed to be pushing Stella's tolerance as it challenged her world in which men were seen as being perpetrators of her abuse. Tensions were prominent around Geoffrey's wish to have a sexual relationship. Stella was happy to remain as friends, living in separate accommodation. She wanted to continue in this relationship if it remained platonic. It seemed as though Stella was at a choice point in her life as to how important this relationship was to her. Her life was relatively stable up to this point, and she enjoyed the company of a circle of female friends visiting. She talked about wanting a relationship with a boyfriend and to become a mother one day, but not currently. Stella was afraid of losing her relationship while she deliberated on what she wanted for her adult life and finally agreed that Geoffrey could move in with her. Soon after he moved in, she told me she had thoughts of worthlessness that she hadn't had for some time and periods of 'losing time', when she was lost in thought about the past, with memories of her childhood abuse re-emerging.

After six supportive counselling sessions in which we focused on Stella's adult relationship and what she wished to do (allow her partner to move in or live apart), she decided that she did not wish for Geoffrey to move in as she found she was feeling out of control with her life when he was staying with her. She decided to tell him this, and that she wished the relationship to continue but not as a live-in partnership. Stella told me that she loved Geoffrey, and, if he loved her, he would wait until she was ready.

Couple session

At Stella's request, I had a session to support her through telling her partner about what she wished to do with the relationship in terms of living independently at this point in time. Geoffrey talked about his awareness that she was increasingly unwell as their relationship moved into being closer and they discussed increasing the physical intimacy in their relationship. This conversation heralded Stella's retreat into the past and the past abuse, which she had discussed with him. He was prepared to continue in a relationship in which he maintained his own home and spent time with Stella at her flat, which was an arrangement that worked for Stella. They both were in their own therapy programmes with the mental health services again by this stage and so realised that they were each on parallel but different healing paths after dealing with early traumatic backgrounds. Geoffrey had had a brother who had drowned in a swimming accident when Geoffrey was only ten years old, and his traumatic death had affected Geoffrey throughout his life since.

On the understanding they would remain platonic friends who lived separately, Stella continued to maintain an independent life with Geoffrey. She allowed more time within it to socialise with Geoffrey more gradually, so that the friendship could develop more fully. I suggested that they might periodically review their future goals with a couple therapist as time went on and challenges from the past arose for each of them, making relating to one another difficult. They agreed with this plan, and we left our contact at this point, with Stella returning to a women's support group for survivors of childhood sexual abuse.

Reflection on the case study of Stella

In the case study of Stella, the findings of Canton-Corte et al.'s (2015) study are echoed. These researchers examined the effects of secure, avoidant and anxious attachment styles on depressive symptomatology in adult women who had historical CSA. The type of abuse, the relationship with the perpetrator and whether the abuse was continuous or one-off affected the attachment style the researchers discovered. Stella's abuse had been continuous, from the age of five years, and she took more of the abuse in order to protect her younger sister. The depression and anxiety she experienced as an adolescent and adult manifested in a coping style involving bulimic and anorexic behaviours that alternated between binge eating, purging and fasting to the point of maintaining a dangerously low body weight. Her excessive exercising impacting her joints was a consequence of the eating disorder, which had left its legacy as a chronic pain syndrome.

Stella anxiety in attaching to adults also related to her relationship with her mother, the primary attachment figure, who did not believe her disclosure of abuse. This early experience is important in imprinting attachment styles, which can affect every facet of the adult woman's life. Parenting, romantic relationships and the durability of peer and partner relationships can all be impacted by the aftermath of CSA for women survivors. Stella's relationship with her boyfriend, Geoffrey, was raising anxiety about trust and whether he would abandon or mistreat her when they started living together. However, Stella did have the secure base of her lifelong relationship with her aunt, who showed an enduring interest in Stella's and Vaiula's welfare when they were children and through into adolescence and adulthood. Previous research has found that a secure attachment style can be beneficial in disclosure with a parental figure, such as a member of the child's extended family (*whānau*) or *hapu* (subtribe) or *iwi* (tribe). Alternatively, non-disclosure can be the norm owing to a history of colonisation (Braithwaite, 2018). Cultural norms may make the informal adoption of a child more normal and acceptable, which can lessen the impact of the abuse by removing the child from the parental home. The relationship with Aunt Violet acted as a buffering, protective factor in the narrative of Stella and her life throughout adolescence to adulthood.

This secure attachment to the non-offending caregiver can serve to regulate the survivor's negative affect and act as a protective factor to lower anxiety in the face of stressful life events (Wallis & Woodworth, 2021). The present case study mirrors this finding and further suggests that a secure attachment style is not necessarily a protective factor in the development of mental illness, including eating disorders, anxiety and depression, which Canton-Cortes et al. (2015) proposed. In their research, there was no connection made between an avoidant attachment style and depression (Canton-Cortes et al., 2015, p. 433) when the abuse was rated as more severe. Stella's abuse was extensive in terms of time, involving many years of abuse (5–11 years), and the relationship to her perpetrator was close (stepfather), indicative of incest. Her abuse also involved penetration as well as other behaviours including sexual grooming and gang rape by her stepfather's friends, and threats and force were both present.

The relationship with the aunt was the major protective factor in both Stella's and her sister's Vaiula's early upbringing through to adolescence and adulthood. I was aware and pleased to hear that this relationship continued in the background when I was seeing Stella for supportive counselling. Auntie Violet had all of the characteristics of the protective non-offending caregiver conducive to disclosure, as outlined by Wallis and Woodworth, (2021, p. 1). She believed in the children and what they said to her; she asked them specifically about abuse from the stepfather, mentioning what kinds of abuse there could be and asking the sisters if they had experienced any of these behaviours at the hands of their stepfather. Third, Violet's emotional support of the sisters was clear in her decision to offer them an alternative family and home when the child protection services investigated and took them out of their home. She provided a context for their growth and healing after what they had endured for years. Auntie Violet had also supported them through the formal disclosure process once charges were laid with police and the court case that followed. This case was ongoing over some years owing to the charges laid also against the other men who were involved in the sexual abuse of the sisters.

Chenier et al. (2021), in the Canadian context, write of the need for both the authorities and the victims and their caregivers to have ongoing support through the formal disclosure of child sexual abuse in various reporting processes via the criminal justice system. The content analysis of 231 non-institutional cases of child sexual abuse brought against alleged perpetrators showed an attrition rate at numerous junctures in the criminal justice process, with the first attrition happening between the child sexual abuse incident(s) and the initial reporting to police. The authors found that 5–25% of complainants drop off at this point. (Chenier et al., 2021, p. 2). The second point of withdrawal of charges occurred through the investigation process and then referral to the court prosecutor, where reasons for and against the case are heard. Further withdrawal by survivors occurred during the court process (Chenier et al., 2021, p. 2). The historical disclosure of CSA becomes even more difficult for the authorities to investigate when the passage of time changes where perpetrators may be residing, dissociation impacts historical traumatic memory, and witnesses/supporters who knew about the abuse may no longer be living or available (Chenier et al., 2021).

Delayed disclosure is common for the host of reasons mentioned in this chapter, including the availability of a secure relationship with a caregiving adult who believes the survivor and acts to protect her. Fears of upsetting the family, losing the primary wage earner (if the perpetrator is in this role) and forever changing one's family through the act of disclosing can be other contextual factors that lead to decisions not to disclose or to delay disclosure.

The implications for practice

For helping professionals, various therapeutic strategies are recommended when they are working with adult survivors of CSA throughout the life trajectory. Such strategies are seen as building secure therapeutic relationships in which the type and duration of abuse can be assessed safely. Sometimes, inpatient or day-patient stays or a return to existing therapeutic relationships are needed. Stella, for example, returned to a women's therapy group she had previously attended for ongoing support. When suicidality features, it may be inadvisable to explore past trauma until the safety framework is in place, which could involve inpatient treatment or a supportive daily programme. For Stella, when her eating disorder was her primary coping mechanism, treatment of the eating disorder was needed before any traumatic memory work was engaged in, as recommended by Herman (1992).

Trust in the therapeutic relationship may be more difficult to build where the abuse is extensive and ongoing in terms of frequency and duration, when the experience involves close family members as abusers, and when grooming/force, physical abuse or threats of retribution are a part of the perpetrator's pattern. These factors have been found to be compounding and are more likely to impact the survivor's mental health. An assessment of the various risk and protective factors from the woman survivor's past and present life, from her perspective is important in understanding why a telling or a retelling of a historical abuse narrative is needed. For Stella, a new romantic relationship with a boyfriend and the prospect of a long-term commitment to a life partner at some point in the future were tipping the balance of her life. It seemed her daily routine had stabilised in recent years with her move into independent housing and employment. She was able to keep her caregiver employment and maintain a circle of friends. She had been alternating between avoidance and anxious attachment styles in relation to her current boyfriend who was pushing 'too fast' to formalise their relationship by moving into the same flat. Throughout this time, Stella continued to have contact with her aunt with whom she had managed to develop a secure attachment since the abuse with her stepfather was disclosed. This in itself was quite remarkable, given the extent, nature and severity of her abuse.

Assessing the availability of protective caregivers in the extended-family context is a neglected feature in the reviewed risk and resiliency literature on how survivors both find the courage to disclose to another and, ultimately, rebound from CSA as adults. This is likely owing to the way that western societies see the family as being more typically the nuclear formation of parents and children, without referring to extended-family networks or local community elders for support. Cultural factors feature in this wider view of the attachment of children, which needs expansion to aunts, uncles, grandparents and elders in a tribal or local community. The statistics from one study mirror this need to explore a historical family tree going back through the elders who were the originators of family norms. Chenier et al. (2021, p. 7) found that, of those CSA survivors disclosing abuse in their sample in Canada, the vast majority were women (72%), with 99% self-identified as being indigenous to that region, while their perpetrators were largely male (97.4%) and white American, showing a cross-cultural aspect of the abuse. Colonisation and the prevailing cultural dominance of the predominantly

European colonisers over the colonised people (Inuit and native American people), who are the original inhabitants of the land, offer one possible interpretation of such statistics. Survivors having recourse to culturally appropriate helping professionals, police and court workers would seem appropriate to enable such power dynamics to be analysed, alongside the protective factors of being part of an extended family living in the context of a closely knit local community. To support practitioners who work with adult survivors of childhood sexual abuse, cultural safety supervision is recommended in the Aotearoa New Zealand context and in other cultures with a history of colonisation (Social Workers Registration Board, 2013). The context of professional practice in the helping professions in Aotearoa New Zealand acknowledges that Māori (a term acknowledging the traditional owners of the land) are *Tangata Whenua* (the people of the land) (Pack, 2009). *Pakeha* New Zealanders (New Zealanders of European descent) are seen as the *Manuhiri*, or visitors to this country, within the founding document outlining the responsibilities and rights of the two peoples, known as the Treaty of Waitangi.

Cultural safety supervision is a term used to describe a form of consultation and supervision in clinical practice that cultivates an awareness of one's own cultural background and how this influences and shapes one's practice in an ongoing way. In order to develop such a competency, the clinician proactively seeks a supervisor who can guide this continuous reflection and critique of their practice with clients in the context of a culture that is based on the spirit of the Treaty of Waitangi. The Treaty of Waitangi is based on the principles of protection, partnership, self-determination and participation (Pack, 2009, p. 176). Forming and maintaining relationships with clients that are '*mana* enhancing' (acknowledging and supporting indigenous cultural beliefs) are specific requirements of social work practice. Furthermore, a knowledge of culturally appropriate assessment is required for competent practice in Aotearoa New Zealand (Social Workers Registration Board, 2013). This assessment in the case of Stella might involve a family tree of the extended family's village to identify those still living in Western Samoa. The impact of the move for the extended family might be explored and how the absence of grandparents and elders and a local village impacted the family functioning when the nuclear family relocated to New Zealand.

Conclusion

More research is needed into the role of the supportive caregiver in the disclosure of CSA across the lifespan. This relationship has the potential to support the woman CSA survivor who, throughout her adult life, may need to revisit her abuse at many junctures, as the case study of Stella illustrates. Thorough assessment of the risks and protective factors offering buffering against the ongoing effects of the abuse is routinely needed, and the person to whom the survivor disclosed often highlights who these important support people and significant others were and how they continue to feature in the survivor's life. When identified, these relationships are significant also for offering opportunities to process traumatic memory when the safety of a protective other is present.

Where there are professional others in this caregiving role, as there were during Stella's successful treatment for an eating disorder, these individuals may provide a secure base over time if they are still working in the same services. Owing to burn-out and vicarious traumatisation, change in personnel working in the mental health service is a given, and, therefore, clients need to adapt to different workers who occupy the same roles with which they came to feel safe and supported. Addressing the vicarious traumatisation of the workers and obtaining appropriate supervision of practice, including cultural safety supervision, are imperative if the relationship with the survivor client is to be most efficacious.

In terms of services provided for adult survivors in the health care system, with clients who are deeply affected by CSA in an ongoing way, a revolving-door approach is probably the expectation, with re-presentations at key moments likely to be the pattern. These re-presentations need to be anticipated and even planned for across the lifespan, rather than being anticipated as a one-off contact. Stella had a need for continuity of service availability when she wanted to refer back to the community mental health services owing to challenges with her boyfriend. This re-presentation for service in a revolving-door fashion is common to many clients who have a history of childhood sexual abuse, which may not be understood by service managers and their need for capped numbers of sessions under public service funding arrangements.

Finally, the trauma of disclosing to the authorities needs to be better acknowledged and understood in the judicial process. Specifically, how to support women making historical claims of abuse, and the risks of dropout and withdrawal throughout the investigation process need to be part of the education of police and legal professionals. Appropriately trained victim support services need to be available to assist women through the rigorous process involved in remembering their original trauma and bringing it into a public context, which may involve a rekindling of the past.

In the next chapter, we move from the realm of relationships and the role of attachment to that of whether to try for a pregnancy and to have a child. This phase of development can potentially run from menarche through to menopause and involve very complex decisions around contraception, fertility, parenting and finances. We will explore the challenges these stages in development hold for the adult survivor of CSA. As decision making relies on a belief in one's own power and control of one's body, women's most fertile years can throw up a range of challenges that necessitate revisiting former beliefs and involve a retelling of one's personal narrative about how the abuse has impacted one's life choices.

References

Bowlby, J. (1973). *Attachment and Loss. Separation, Anxiety and Anger* (Vol. 2). New York: Basic Books.

Braithwaite, J. (2018). Colonized silence: confronting the colonial link in rural Alaska native survivors' non-disclosure of child sexual abuse. *Journal of Child Sexual Abuse*, 27(6), 589–611. doi:10.1080/10538712.2018.1491914

Briere, J. (1996). *Therapy for Adults Molested as Children: Beyond Survival* (2nd ed., revised and expanded). New York: Springer.

Canton-Cortes, D., Cortes, M. R., & Canton, J. (2015). Child sexual abuse, attachment style, and depression: the role of the characteristics of abuse. *Journal of Interpersonal Violence*, 30(3), 420–436. doi:10.1177/0886260514535101

Chenier, K., Shawyer, A., Williams, A., & Milne, R. (2021). 'Cold feet': the attrition of historic child sexual abuse cases reported to the police in a Northern Canadian territory. *Child Abuse and Neglect*, 120. doi:10.1016/j.chiabu.2021.105206

Domhardt, M., Munzer, A., Fegert, J. M., & Goldbeck, L. (2015). Resilience in survivors of child sexual abuse: a systematic review of the literature. *Trauma, Violence, and Abuse*, 16(4), 476–493. doi:10.1177/1524838014557288

Godbout, N., Briere, J., Sabourin, S., & Lussier, Y. (2014). Child sexual abuse and subsequent relational and personal functioning: the role of parental support. *Child Abuse and Neglect*, 38(2), 317–325.

Hergass, S. (2019). A model of art therapy for Aboriginal children within the preschool. Thesis, Australian Catholic University.

Herman, J. (1992). *Trauma and Recovery*. Basic Books.

Howe, D. (2011). *Attachment across the Life Course: A Brief Introduction* (2nd ed.). Bloomsbury.

Karakurt, G., & Silver, K. E. (2014). Therapy for childhood sexual abuse survivors using attachment and family systems theory orientations. *American Journal of Family Therapy*, 42(1), 79–91. doi:10.1080/01926187.2013.772872

Miller, K. J. (1993). Prevalence and process of disclosure of childhood sexual abuse among eating-disordered women. *Eating Disorders*, 1, 211–225.

Pack, M. (2002). *Sexual Abuse Counsellors' Responses to Trauma and Stress: A Social Work Perspective*. Victoria University of Wellington.

Pack, M. (2004). Sexual abuse counsellors' responses to trauma and stress: a social work perspective. *Journal of New Zealand Association of Counsellors, Te Ropu Kaiwhiriwhiri o Aotearoa*, 25(2), 1–17.

Pack, M. (2009). Social work (adult). In K. Grimmer-Somers & G. Nehrenz (Eds.), *Practical Tips in Finding the Evidence: An Allied Health Primer* (pp. 176–199). Manila, Philippines: UST.

Social Workers Registration Board. (2013). *Ngā Paerewa Kaiakatanga Matua – Core Competence Standards*. New Zealand: Social Workers Registration Board.

Wallis, C. R. D., & Woodworth, M. (2021). Non-offending caregiver support in cases of child sexual abuse: an examination of the impact of support on formal disclosures. *Child Abuse and Neglect*, 113. doi:10.1016/j.chiabu.2021.104929

Winnicott, D. (1965). *The Maturational Processes and the Facilitating Environment*. Hogarth Press and the Institute of Psychoanalysis.

4 Education, work, pregnancy and parenting

> She was only 8. He was in his 20s. Sameera Qureshi didn't fully understand that she'd been assaulted by this distant relative, a Muslim just like her, until two decades later when she became a sexual health educator and started teaching students in schools about sexual abuse.
>
> 'I was 30 years old when I realized I am a survivor,' said Qureshi, now 36, speaking at a panel titled, '#MeToo in Sacred Spaces,' in Columbus, Ohio, in September. 'I can reflect back, and now all the traumatic memories start to make sense. My body … has kept the score till this day as I continue to unravel and work through the trauma that my body has held for that many years.'
>
> (Hatuqa, 2018)

Introduction

In the quote above, Sameer Quereshi discusses the personal background that motivated her intense interest in working as a sexual health educator, fuelled by her experience of CSA (Hatuqa, 2018). Common to many women survivors of CSA, recognition of the after-effects of abuse may not be acknowledged until much later, with CSA recollections and issues often arising in early adulthood (Alaggia, 2005; Alaggia et al., 2019). What is remembered initially may not be thought of as being 'sexual abuse'. It is not until the perpetrator's behaviour is reflected on and understood from an adult perspective that the recognition dawns and decisions about disclosure are faced. When family members are involved in the abuse and the survivor was a child when the CSA occurred, there is an inevitable violation of trust. This betrayal can come from the family members either minimising the abuse or denying that it happened and/or from a family member being the perpetrator of the abuse. Protecting the perpetrator, who may be seen as the head of the family or primary breadwinner, may be a priority for the survival of the family as a unit. The depth of the survivor's realisation as an adult may bring with it, into the foreground, the rekindling of the initial betrayal of trust. Such flashpoints can create a crisis, and this disruption of everyday life can be particularly distressing for the adult survivor who may attempt to disclose in an iterative way to a professional helper, partner or significant other.

DOI: 10.4324/9781032669205-4

The quality of the woman survivor's experience of her parental and family relationships can affect her own subsequent parenting or relationship with her partner and her own children, as we have seen in the previous chapter with its focus on attachment styles. Such experiences in partnership and parenting will be explored in this chapter in relation to decisions to parent or to avoid relationships and parenting. Experiences of engaging with teaching and learning and subsequent work will also be highlighted, as these key themes also dominate this phase of life as survivors prepare for their future work roles. It is in this phase of life (20s–30s) that women most often complete higher learning and education in preparation for a career, whether this be paid employment, or full-time or part-time employment in combination with parenting. Experiences of forging couple relationships are a feature of this age range, and it can be the first time that issues relating to a history of CSA can emerge. The parallel issues of coercive factors in adult partnerships may be recognised as an ongoing pattern of abuse, and the need for change in a woman survivor's narrative may be highlighted.

Themes from the research literature: women survivors in their 20s and 30s

There are several themes in the literature as to why women delay telling anyone about their abuse until they are aged in their 20s and 30s. These themes include the blaming of women because of societal beliefs and the internalised self-blame of women. Second, underlying family dynamics can be an ongoing barrier to disclosure of CSA; and, third, there can be ambivalence caused by fears about the effects of disclosure on family and significant others.

During this phase, there is usually greater individuation from one's family of origin in an attempt to create new adult relationships and an independent identity in the world. As the preceding chapters have illustrated, the first relationships we experience are strongly influenced by the relationships we have developed in nuclear and extended family systems through the process of interaction with caregivers and the dynamic of attachment. As discussed in Chapter Three, lack of caregiver support may inhibit disclosure of CSA until these years of young adulthood (Wallis & Woodworth, 2021). Conversely, if there is caregiver or other support, this may act as a protective relationship that continues to be a feature of the ongoing need for disclosure of CSA as the child grows into an adolescent and young adult (Guyon et al., 2021).

Blaming the victim and self-blame

Women survivors are often found to avoid disclosure owing to believing that they are responsible for bringing the abuse on themselves. Later, they can internalise this belief and are subject to being blamed by others for what has occurred (Alaggia, 2005; Alaggia et al., 2019). This tendency for blaming the victim to turn into self-blame is accounted for in various ways. Many taking a feminist view towards the disclosure of CSA see it as being related to women's position in a patriarchal society (Alaggia et al., 2019). Women's position is traditionally considered to be more often in subordinate roles from a feminist perspective. From this positioning, societal beliefs tend to blame women for being provocative in various ways, including by their dress and behaviour. This gendered analysis of disclosure can be seen more broadly alongside other gender-related myths about women, deflecting attention from the perpetrator who most often is male (Alaggia et al., 2019).

These themes mirror the findings of a literature review that identified the positive and negative responses following the disclosure of CSA when the disclosure involved significant others. The authors reported the impact on the survivor of the telling of their story of CSA and the subsequent aftermath for those confided in by the survivor (Tener & Murphy, 2015). Survivors of CSA told researchers that it was helpful if those who were disclosed to remained emotionally calm during the disclosure and supportively allowed them to discuss what happened to allow them to integrate memories of CSA over time. Negative responses to disclosure were found to minimise the abuse, telling the survivor to move on from it and refusing to engage in further discussion about it (Tener & Murphy, 2015).When there was a strong reaction against the perpetrator and anger expressed towards the perpetrator, women most often tended to close down the disclosure and delay further disclosure based on the negative experience of telling, as they felt the person disclosed to was no longer listening to them (Tener & Murphy, 2015).

Ambivalence about disclosure and 're-authoring'

Ambivalence about disclosure of CSA is common when relationships within the family are tentative and untrusting, when the costs of disclosure are high and when the non-offending parent or caregiver is ambivalent/preoccupied in their attachment to their children (Bolen & Lamb, 2004). Ambivalence may also be both a precursor to and an effect of the traumatic experience of the disclosure for the non-offending parent or guardian (Bolen & Lamb, 2004). These interactions can influence the subsequent ways that women survivors who have experienced abuse relate to primary attachment figure(s). These issues of ambivalence in relating can be a feature of survivors' relationships throughout the life course. Narrative models of family therapy, such as those developed by the foundational work of Epston and White (1992), developed a framework for understanding how family systems operate to create and promote problems as well as associating individual family members with problems. When a family member was defined as being 'the problem', they were found to be operating from wider family beliefs and did not have the detachment to see how they had become imbued with the family's problem-saturated narratives that were not of their own making. Some brands of family therapy worked to look at each member's understanding of the 'problem' as a means of demonstrating the authoring of problems and to refocus the family on the idea that 'the problem is the problem'. This understanding of 're-authoring' narratives provided the stigmatised family member with a chance to transcend the invitation to be labelled by others as being 'the problem' (Epston & White, 1992; White, 1995).

When child sexual abuse is disclosed during adulthood by women survivors, they are often blamed for what can be a dysfunctional series of affective ties within a family, leading to a vulnerability to being targeted by perpetrators from within or without the *whānau*, or extended family. While much time was given to blaming the mother for not providing the secure base for the child who was abused, the focus has since moved to providing help to the identified victim and assistance to the adult caregivers within a family to improve the whole extended family system.

Increasingly, attention in research has been focused on how adult women come to understand they have been sexually abused in childhood, leading to disclosure of a formal or informal nature. Until the child comes to understand that the behaviour of the perpetrator was abusive, disclosure is unlikely to be made, as the child normalises or gives some alternative explanation for the behaviour of the perpetrator. It is often when the young person leaves home to go and live independently from family and/or to begin study at university that they come to realise the enormity of what has happened earlier in life. It is this gradual dawning of having been a victim of CSA and realisation of its manifold, long-lasting effects that we will go on to explore in the following section.

How adult survivors of CSA come to understand they have been abused

It is now considered that there is an identifiable process underlying the pathway by which adult women are thought to reach an understanding that they have been sexually abused as children. The aim of one Norwegian study was to explore how adult women over the age of 18 came to understand the perpetrator's behaviour as sexual abuse. In Norway, there were police campaigns following the #MeToo movement encouraging women to report suspicions of abuse of children in the large city setting (Halvorsen et al., 2020, p. 207). The average age of the participants who came forward was 36 years old. A semi-structured interview schedule asked participants about their process of realising their perpetrator's behaviour was sexual abuse by allowing participants to tell their story in their own way, keeping a focus on understanding the process of disclosure. From a thematic analysis of the transcribed interviews, the understanding of what had occurred was a gradual awakening, triggered by flashbacks, body sensations and current relationships as adults.

Stige et al. (2020) discovered what the contributing factors were in this process of coming to terms with emerging experiences later to be considered to be CSA. As in this book, the WHO (2017) definition of CSA was used. The WHO definition of sexual abuse is sexual activity that is inappropriate in that a child can neither comprehend nor consent to it owing to age and stage (Stige et al., 2020, p. 206). In line with Herman's (1992; Herman, 2015) theorising, it mentions the double bind of the child depending on the perpetrator as the primary attachment figure while knowing that the same figure is inflicting pain and distress on them. This double bind of needing care and trying to avoid the hurt inflicted by the abuse creates an insoluble dilemma for the child (Halvorsen et al., 2020, p. 206).

From a thematic analysis of the transcribed interviews, the understanding of what had occurred was pieced together from fragments of memory made available as spontaneous flashbacks or dreams and/or life themes triggered by current relationship issues and various body sensations during sex, pregnancy and birth. These experiences were found helpful for the survivor to coalesce the shards of experience to form a coherent whole over time. This was particularly so when the woman attended therapy that enabled the experience to be viewed more chronologically. This assisted the woman to assemble a personal narrative, with the self being the actor throughout the narrative (Halvorsen et al., 2020, pp. 211–214).

Some of the women survivors who were interviewed described pushing memories away. This often led to nightmares and dissociated states that were identified as involving fragmented identities. Chronological memories were often unavailable, as the following participant explains:

> I had this alter ego, and she had been through a lot too, so I have always struggled a lot with nightmares. But I think it was in grade eight that the nightmares got worse, which turned out to be flashback nightmares. But at that time, I was afraid of losing it, because I didn't quite get that it was my memories. So now I got them [memories] because I have put them in the right place.
>
> (Halvorsen et al., 2020, p. 211)

In the following case study, the support of the parents in helping their adolescent to recognise sexually coercive/grooming behaviours by an older man was important to disclosure of the abuse. The man's behaviour as a family friend went unrecognised by the adolescent, while her mother, who observed the relationship, enabled her daughter to see that the age, power imbalance, and her relative naïveté meant the relationship was itself abusive.

Case study 1: Renee

Renee, a 20-year-old university student of French descent, presented to our pregnancy and grief and loss clinic with an unwanted pregnancy for which she sought pre-decision counselling over what to do next. She attended with her mother as support person, and her mother explained some of the context and background to the pregnancy.

Renee had befriended a fellow classmate who had taken her home to meet her family, who were from South America, having recently relocated to New Zealand looking for a 'better life'. An older brother, Juan, who was 30 years old, used to 'hang out' and spend time with Renee and her girlfriend, to the extent that Renee saw her friend's brother as a brother figure owing to his relationship with the two of them.

Renee's mother explained that Renee had been diagnosed with Asperger's syndrome and ADHD (Attention Deficit Hyperactivity Disorder) as a 13 year old, so found expressing herself to be very difficult. Socially, she was developmentally delayed, leading to a vulnerability to acquiescing to the wishes of others. In school reports, it was noted by her teachers that there were learning difficulties that made it hard for her to communicate with her teachers and classmates clearly. Renee's mother further explained that she believed that, because of his age, the brother of her classmate (Juan) had groomed Renee for sexual contact within the emotional intimacy of her relationship with his sister, who was her best friend. The context of having a best friend who was trusting had been good for Renee as she was able to confide in her girlfriend and socialise with her.

When she first presented to see me as counsellor, Renee was ambivalent about the pregnancy. This ambivalence was due to the relationship with her best friend and her friend's brother (Juan). She did not want to 'cause trouble' for Juan but was clear that she did not want to have a baby after a first sexual experience and was confused about the relationship with her friend's brother.

The clinical team assessed coercive factors present in the relationship owing to age and also Renee's diagnosis of Asperger's syndrome, making her vulnerable to misreading interpersonal behaviour accurately – in other words, to be unable to intuit the motives of others, including predatory adult male advances. Therefore, she could not see these themes owing to looking through the eyes of a pre-teen because of her Asperger's and ADHD, with limited life experience and social finesse in interpersonal situations. Her mother recounted in interview an earlier incident at 13 years. Renee had been 'groped' by a middle-aged male customer when she was shopping in a department store. She had told her mother after the event but did not interpret what had happened as being sexual abuse. The perpetrator of her earlier abuse fled, and so no further action had been taken. Renee had had a term off school as she was fearful of leaving the house after that incident, so was referred to correspondence school for a semester and received counselling from a psychologist. She returned to a different school, closer to home, the next year. The incident with Juan, while consensual from Renee's perspective, was located in the context of a trusting friendship with her girlfriend. His sexual advances had retriggered some of the issues for Renee from the earlier incident of sexual molestation by the stranger in the department store. Renee described feeling anxious and powerless to demand that Juan use a condom. He reassured her that there was no likelihood of a pregnancy and, if there was a pregnancy, they could obtain the emergency contraceptive pill. Renee was not able to see a pattern of being victim of unwanted sexualised contact by older men. However, she did reflect on the fact that she did not wish to leave her current schooling, which would have been a likely consequence of continuing the pregnancy.

Renee's parents had made a complaint to the police, who were investigating the allegations made, and, therefore, the police had interviewed Renee. Juan had denied having a sexual relationship at all. While we looked at options with Renee, she very clearly articulated that she did not want to have a baby at that time. With her parents' and health care professionals' support, she was scheduled for a termination of pregnancy, which was completed the next day without complication.

At the follow-up appointment post-procedure, Renee was pleased to be back at university without a break so that she was able to study for her forthcoming exams. She was somewhat sad about the loss of friendship with her girlfriend but aware of her parent's support of her.

Reflections on the case of Renee

If the teen or young person has parents or caregivers who acknowledge the behaviours of the perpetrator as being sexual abuse, this increases the probability of disclosure for this demographic (Guyon et al., 2021). A strong primary attachment to her mother had led to Renee telling her what had happened, in both the current and past episodes of abuse. It was difficult for Renee to see a pattern between the molestation she experienced at the hands of a stranger in a department store as a 13 year old and being groomed for sex by an older brother of her best friend. The primary attachment to her mother enabled disclosure about both his behaviour and the subsequent pregnancy. The case exemplifies how parental reactions to disclosure are critical as they can determine how soon the victim gets help in terms of therapy and appropriate health care. Leaving the pregnancy beyond the point where she had the option of abortion would have had life-changing consequences. The parents were able to provide the context for why the relationship was coercive and abusive.

The 'double bind' of wanting to keep the relationship with her best girlfriend while declining the relationship with her friend's brother can be seen as being related to the phase of life. In later adolescence through to young adulthood, developing and maintaining peer relationships are of paramount importance. Her attachment to her parents as primary attachment figures is prominent at this stage in her life as she was living with them at home as a first-year university student for financial reasons. The mother held the continuity of the two events (the molestation at age 13 years and the knowledge of Renee's vulnerability to being taken advantage of sexually by others). Her mother understood this vulnerability to be due to the earlier developmental delays common to many women with ADHD and Asperger's syndrome. These diagnoses meant that Renee would not see or navigate complex human relationships easily.

For Renee, her awareness was a pathway to understanding why she felt she could not deal with the pregnancy. She was aware that the pregnancy had been the product of a relationship that had moved 'too fast', leaving her little time for reflection on what she wanted. She mentioned 'not being ready' for either the relationship or the pregnancy and now wanted both to 'go away' so she could resume her usual life, at home with her parents and focusing on her studies. This wish for her future life and the reality of an unplanned and unwanted pregnancy that would result in having a baby and being a single parent formed the 'prompt' to informal disclosure to her parents. Her parents facilitated the formal disclosure to the police for investigation.

The effects of disclosure on educational opportunities and career are highlighted by the case study of Renee. When CSA is in the background, yet to be acknowledged, many survivors drop out of education, which has implications for subsequent career, income and quality of life. Alternatively, some survivors go on to have poor experiences of the educational context owing to mental health concerns such as anxiety, insomnia, depression and dissociation, all of which are common symptoms of complex traumatic responses. Disclosure of CSA by women can be a protective factor when disclosure is made in the context of a supportive partner relationship, as the following review of literature attests.

Disclosure of CSA by women and the implications for adult romantic relationships

Studies evaluating the impact of disclosures of CSA on adult romantic relationships are infrequent. Most studies find participants who disclose CSA to their romantic partners have a positive or helpful response. De Montigny Gauthier et al. (2019) interviewed 70 couples where CSA was disclosed to the romantic partner. The most common responses from the romantic partner were reported to be emotional support (94.3%) followed by practical aid (67.1%). A minority of participants (14.3%) reported feeling blamed during the disclosure. To be eligible to participate in the study, couples needed to be aged 18 years or older, to be in a relationship of six months or more and not currently pregnant. Relationship and sexual satisfaction scales were used to indicate the correlation, if any, between disclosure within the relationship and relationship and sexual satisfaction. The findings indicated that survivor-perceived partner responses to disclosure of CSA were associated with both sexual and relationship satisfaction as a couple (de Montigny Gauthier et al., 2019, pp. 485–490).

This research suggests that practitioners need to assess the effects of partner responses to disclosure of CSA carefully. If it is hypothesised that there is likely to be a negative reaction from a partner to a survivor's disclosure of CSA then preparation of the client to decide whether or not they wish to disclose may be needed. If the survivor's estimation of how disclosure will likely be received by those significant others around them is unknown, then it may be helpful to have disclosure of CSA facilitated in the context of therapy. This facilitated disclosure with partners or other significant others ensures that the aftermath of disclosure and any impact on the emotional well-being of the woman survivor can be managed in the therapeutic relationship and any fallout can be processed. Specifically, any anticipated blaming and stigmatising responses from significant others need to be assessed and foreshadowed in a preparatory space, as negative impacts from disclosure have been found to be among the most detrimental to the woman survivor and her healing from CSA (Guyon et al., 2021).

In the event of any anticipated strong reaction from the woman's romantic partner, the therapist or helping professional disclosed to becomes the alternative support person or transitional support figure until the partner comes to terms with the disclosure. Time is sometimes needed if the partner is to process the news of the woman's CSA in order that they are available to offer support while being able to modulate and at times bracket their own anger at how the CSA has impacted the woman's life, including the couple relationship. The partner or significant others may be assisted to seek separate therapy for their issues, which might be quite different from the woman survivor's issues. Often, couple counselling is recommended, involving another therapist to keep the boundaries clear between what is disclosed to the women's individual therapist.

Relational difficulties connected to historical CSA are often disclosed to those involved in general health care as well as to those in the therapeutic context. For one woman survivor of CSA with whom I worked as a mental health professional, the recurring pattern of abuse in subsequent relationships were highlighted. Kayla, a woman aged in her late 20s, presented to the community health agency, referred by her general practitioner with depression and ongoing difficulties with self-harming attempts. The theme of increasingly finding the observer within, who notices patterns in her relating to others, was precipitating a crisis for her. She began to have insight about the reasons for having difficulties relating to others. After being sexually abused at age 12 years when she was raped by an acquaintance, Kayla noticed that, when her supportive relationships became close, she pushed them away. Then she found herself in subsequent relationships that were abusive psychologically, sexually and physically but remained attracted to those partners and those relationships.

Case study 2: Kayla

Kayla is a 28-year-old first-generation New Zealander of Irish origins who presented to mental health services with persistent suicidal ideation. She described having 'always low self-esteem' and appeared anxious, eager to please others and tearful when the acute mental health services were called by her parents. The crisis mobile mental health team paid a home visit owing to this call-out in an apparent emergency. At first assessment, she discussed always wanting to have children and said that she was afraid that she would never have a boyfriend or offspring. Her first sexual experience at age 12 was being raped by a boyfriend. It was from this assault that she contracted the HSV virus, or genital herpes. She said that subsequent to contracting genital herpes she had felt deeply embarrassed. It was a recurring physical reminder of the rape.

She discussed believing in subsequent relationships that she wouldn't get the love she so desired, thus staying in emotionally abusive relationships 'too long' in retrospect. She described a descent into guilt and shame about her CSA whenever a subsequent relationship turned out to be abusive and resulted in her leaving. Kayla described how her subsequent abuse as an adult had included her partners being unfaithful towards her, which she found out sometimes years later. In the most recent partnership, lasting a year, unbeknownst to her, her partner psychologically abused her by taking and sharing naked photos of her and uploading these to social media sites. When Kayla presented to mental health services, she described herself as currently feeling unsafe and suicidal following discovery of the photographs on social media with derogatory responses from her now ex-partner. This discovery led to her decision to make an abrupt end to the relationship after a year of living together. He had asked for an 'open relationship' in which they could each have other partners but continue to live together. This arrangement was unacceptable to Kayla who longed for commitment and fidelity in a relationship. She said she 'still loved him' despite his 'betrayal' of her.

When Kayla was seen acutely, she said she was regretting her decision to leave the abusive partner (Tony). She discussed how she felt pressured into making the decision to end her relationship by her psychologist, parents and girlfriend. She described seeing a psychotherapist intermittently for long-term psychotherapy since the rape at age 12 years and said that she would be seeing her psychologist again in a few weeks. She told me that she had moved home to live with her parents, who knew about the earlier rape and subsequent abuse in her relationship. Moving back to live with her parents was something Kayla thought she would never do. She said that made her feel that she was a 'failure' in her adult life for not being in an independent living situation. She never told them about the difficulties in her adult partnerships as she felt her parents became critical of her for being, once again, in another abusive relationship and having to leave. She described this experience of cutting herself off from her parents and supporters owing to self-blame and wanting to avoid 'I-told-you-so' responses. Kayla visualised herself 'going down the shame drain' in relation to this recurring pattern of guilt at the break-up of her relationships.

Kayla worked in a call centre when she was seen. She discussed being 'sick and tired' of her job, which involved assisting women to leave their abusive relationships and seek refuge housing. In this job, she was doing what Sameera did in her career choice – unconsciously entering a field that raised parallel issues to her own abuse. Kayla was assisting women who had been abused in her work when she was unaware of the connection of her career choice to the legacy of her own CSA. Her CSA seemed to be ignited by the traumatic material she encountered daily in her work role. The potential for vicarious traumatisation was unrecognised and so was unacknowledged. She thought that motherhood might be an alternative career but, without a partner, she realised she could not fulfil this dream as she would only have her family for practical, financial and emotional support. She said she wanted to avoid being beholden to them for the reasons earlier mentioned.

Kayla told me she was currently having fleeting suicidal ideation, with no clear plan of harming herself, in the context of her relationship loss. She told the emergency mental health helpline that she 'wouldn't be here' when they asked her about follow-up appointment times with the mental health team. Kayla had been so down after her relationship ended that she described wanting to end her life but could not say this more clearly and so had minimised the way she was feeling and had internalised her feelings instead. She admitted that she couldn't be relied on to keep herself safe when I asked her this question directly. Kayla then disclosed that she had attempted an overdose on Panadol about one week earlier but, fortunately, had disclosed to her parents who intervened and took her to the emergency room for medical attention.

A psychotherapeutic-orientated approach rather than medication was recommended by the multidisciplinary team, and so I saw her initially over a six-week period on a weekly basis, with the understanding that she would return to her psychologist at the end of our contact for the ongoing psychotherapy. In the review at the end of the six weeks of seeing Kayla weekly for supportive counselling, she stated that all had been going a bit better for her. There had been no attempts at self-harm, and her parents regularly checked in with her about how she was feeling. She ended up contacting her ex-boyfriend's mother to tell her everything that had transpired, including pressure from him to have an open relationship. She described the disclosure of CSA at age 12 to her mother-in-law as 'a release' for her, and the mother-in-law seemed very supportive of Kayla. Through her remaining supportive towards Kayla and expressing disappointment in her son, Kayla felt heard and validated. Kayla stated that they had planned a family meeting for the following week with the three of them, once Tony's mother had spoken with him. Kayla stated that, even if she never saw her boyfriend again after the planned family discussion, at least the weight of his behaviour would be 'off her chest'. For the rest of the evening, she told me, she had plans to get together with a few friends. She would continue with her work in the call centre as she thought about what she wanted to do in terms of career and retraining. For the meantime, she would return to her psychologist for ongoing therapy.

Reflections on the case study of Kayla

Adult women's experiences of CSA can rekindle a recurrent pattern of shame in their experience of their adult relationships. It is as though their trust in the past partnerships is betrayed again by the recent partner, echoing the original CSA. Shame in adulthood following CSA is an under-researched area of the literature, meaning that the voices of survivors and their lived experience are sometimes missing from discussion of the process of disclosure of CSA. A recent scoping review of survivors' experiences of shame in adulthood found that shame can impede the process of disclosure of CSA across the life course

(MacGinley et al., 2019). Twenty-eight peer-reviewed studies were analysed to investigate common themes in the lived experience of survivors. It was found that the survivors' experience of shame predicted both dissociation and re-victimisation in adult relationships (MacGinley et al., 2019, p. 1141). As we have seen in previous chapters, attachment and connection to others significantly assist disclosure. Therefore, if there is the quality of relationship that facilitates disclosure and supports the ongoing healing of the adult survivor, the relationship can be a framework for recovery. Conversely, if there is a negative or shame-inducing response from those disclosed to, the potential for disconnection and isolation is heightened. In this regard, the earlier-mentioned psychological difficulties and mental health diagnoses can more often be a feature of this social disconnection and ongoing impact of shame on the survivor's sense of self and efficacy in the world (MacGinley et al., 2019, p. 1142). Shame may act as an ongoing obstacle to disclosure, so reducing the survivor's ability to reach out for help by connecting with others.

This process of shame leading to social withdrawal and a diminished sense of self I have conceptualised as a spiralling process by which the self becomes enmeshed with the lived experience of shame. As a consequence, shame can, at times, become all-encompassing. The sense of shame promotes a vocal inner critic who works to erode negatively the survivor's feelings of esteem and worthiness (MacGinley et al., 2019, pp. 1142–1143). The process of CSA recovery from the helping practitioners' perspective often involves highlighting the self-defeating process of self-blame as a way of raising self-awareness of the process. With an awareness of this reccurring pattern, the woman survivor can be encouraged to sit back and observe and gently challenge the inner critic to disrupt the internal monologue of shame and self-blame. The act of disclosure of one's abuse to a trusted adult can, if met with support, shift the internalised sense of shame. Educating women about the shame–self-blame spiral can be one way of liberating women to reach out to others and improve recovery opportunities through sustaining relationships. Increasing self-compassion is ultimately the goal of such psychosocial interventions with survivors. What Kayla referred to as 'going down the shame drain', which resulted in negative self-talk fuelled by feelings of unworthiness, can be reframed, once the low point or crisis of suicidality and self-harm has passed and some sense of normalcy returns.

Shame and self-stigmatisation as a process hampering disclosure

Although experiences of embarrassment or shame are common in adolescence or when adults face a new socially charged relational experience, such as asking a friend out on a date or having a romantic proposal rejected, such situations are considered part of the learning of social mores in a new or socially constructed situation where boundaries and one's understanding of appropriate behaviour are tested. As MacGinley et al. (2019) theorise, where trauma is a feature of this experience, shame can act as a protective mechanism, sending an alert to our self that something is wrong and a boundary has been transgressed. Seen in this way, the self has been compromised in some respect by our own actions or by the actions of another when shame features. Thus, shame has been established during interaction with another and is shaped by and in the relationship (MacGinley et al., 2019, pp. 136–137). The experience of shame is considered to be subjective and unique to the individual who goes through it. Consequently, experiences of shame may differ from person to person, with some having shame triggered more easily by a harsh internal critic or the internalised voice of a critical parent or authority figure that has been established earlier in life (MacGinley et al., 2019, pp. 136–137).

When shame has been ongoing as a subjective response to events over many years, such as following early abuse experiences, it can become a reccurring pattern that impacts the survivor's sense of self. There can be a tendency to wither and withdraw when shame is felt, which increases the feelings of disconnection from others and results in social isolation. Thus, Stella's withdrawal from her mother when she was disbelieved about her CSA led to a coping mechanism of withdrawing or retaliating owing to feeling shame about her behaviour as she was growing up. Her subsequent experiences of withdrawing during her relationship with her boyfriend, Geoffrey, reinforced this self-protective strategy. Some theorists differentiate guilt from shame; as MacGinley et al. (2019) summarise, the conceptual distinction is that guilt means I have done something wrong, while shame says 'I am wrong' (MacGinley et al., 2019). Taken together, guilt and shame can lead to a self-stigmatising cycle that can potentially spiral upwards and downwards, depending on how the survivor experiences subjectively what is happening to her both at the time and, as an adult, looking back at what happened in childhood. This shame–self-stigmatisation cycle influences the decision making to disclose to another or not to disclose.

If a survivor of CSA, as an adult, has this internalised sense of an unworthy or in some way inadequate self, it is very unlikely that they will feel a sense of agency to report their abuse or disclose it to anyone. Daily acts of resistance to abuse, particularly when power and control feature, may helpfully involve withdrawal from relationships, but this in turn can act to fuel and empower the perpetrator to continue to abuse.

In summary, externalising shame through disclosure of CSA to a helping professional or significant other can create the impetus for an upward spiral. Disclosure with a trained therapist or helping professional is a starting point to identify what is occurring when feelings of unworthiness lead to thoughts of self-harm proliferating. In particular, disclosure of one's abuse and the process of guilt and self-blame that can be triggered can be a starting point to educate the survivor about the dynamic of what I have called the 'self-stigmatisation spiral', which I have conceptualised as the process for women survivors of CSA in the diagram in Figure 4.1.

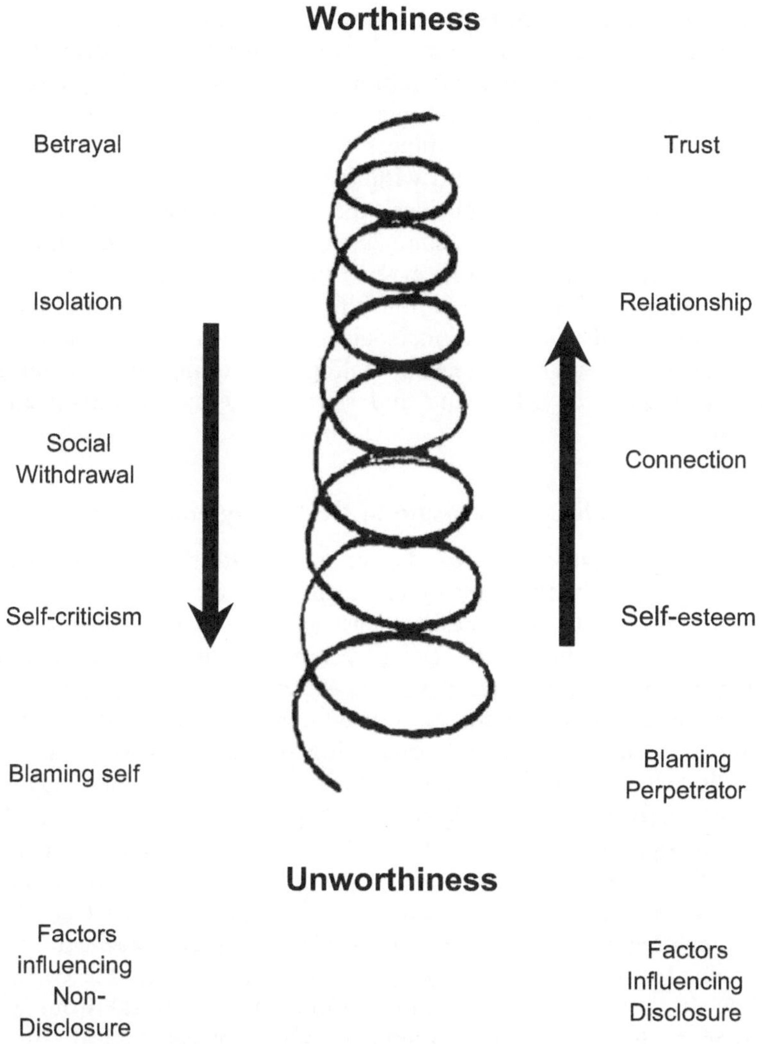

Figure 4.1 The Self-Stigmatisation–Shame Spiral

This diagram depicts the role of disclosure as a dynamic springboard for moderating shame that is generated by negative responses from others and the attitudes held by society at large. This chorus of voices is often joined by a self-stigmatising process in which the victim begins to blame herself. This I have conceptualised as the voice of 'the internal critic'. Again, the protective factors of supportive social networks and positive experiences of disclosure can create the safe space characterised by the relational holding of the therapeutic relationship until an 'upward spiral' is created.

Ultimately, the helping professional's aim in continuing to see the woman survivor is to provide a positive experience of disclosure by demonstrating genuine interest, belief and validation of the survivor's process and experience. This is where the dynamic of the 'upward spiral' is evidenced. Likewise, if there are life circumstances that trigger the shaming process, a downward spiral may be engaged with.

The hope is that, in time, this positive experience of disclosure being witnessed and validated might offset the self-stigmatising. Through connection and a relationship in which the disclosure is revisited in the presence of the person who hears and acknowledges, this relationship can guard against the tendency towards shame, self-stigmatisation, social withdrawal and isolation. This connectedness can lead to increasing feelings of valuing the self, offsetting the pervasive sense of self-blame and shame and increasing esteem and worthiness.

The relationship between disclosure of CSA, pregnancy and birth

The psychological pain of CSA can be connected with the physical sensations of the body and can be triggered by the normal physical changes experienced by women during such milestones as menstruation, sex, pregnancy and birth. Such flashpoints can emerge as a crisis, evoking a need for the woman to tell or retell her story of abuse and how it has affected her life across time. Some researchers have found that the body produces signs and bodily symptoms that bring women to health and counselling professionals as an alternative form of disclosure to verbal disclosure (Stige et al., 2020). This body awareness and its associated bodily signs and symptoms are sometimes a clue to CSA. These signs may be indicative of how CSA is currently impacting a woman's life and has impacted it in the past. Recognition of the connection between CSA and the body can occur when in the presence of a trusted other. Body feelings reminiscent of some aspect of the original abuse can trigger a choice point to disclose or to disclose again. For example, the community mental health service I was working within had a referral from a local gynaecologist who was unable to conduct a routine gynaecological assessment of the patient. The difficulties prompting the referral were related to the woman patient being unable to relax enough for a speculum to be introduced during a routine gynaecological examination. Through relaxation training with one of the therapists at our community mental health centre, she was able to discuss an experience of being abused by an older brother from the age of eight. She had never told anyone about the abuse because he had threatened that her disclosure would 'tear the family apart'. When she did tell her parents, they minimised the abuse by saying it was 'normal to experiment'. Though the abuse stopped soon after that, she had internalised a fear of having damaged her family and turned responsibility for the abuse on herself. She had led a solitary life since reaching adulthood, avoiding most relationships. Now, at the age of 29 years, she was at a crossroads, deciding whether she wanted partnership to feature in her life or whether she wanted to remain single and living on her own. The internal examination by the gynaecologist had been requested by her general practitioner's nurse who had difficulty conducting a routine cervical smear, hence the search for answers. Fortunately, with psychotherapy, she was able, in time, to have her regular gynaecological health checks.

In a similar way, Stige et al. (2020, p. 212) record the experience of one of their 30-year-old women research participants who was interviewed for their research. She told the researcher how her body told her when it was time to reconnect with her abuse memories:

> It was just like, it is the strangest thing. As my self-esteem gets into place, now that I can start to like myself and love myself, it was just as if the body said: 'OK, now you are ready to remember', because if it had come earlier I don't think I would had been here today.

Owens et al. (2021) recommend that all health care workers, and especially those who work in the field of women's health, such as nurses, obstetricians and gynaecologists, treat all patients as sexual abuse survivors (Owens et al., 2021, p. 1). The authors, as medical doctors and medical researchers, advocate that all clinicians providing reproductive health care need to have a framework for trauma-informed care, acknowledging the pervasive nature of sexual abuse trauma for women in their care (Owens et al., 2021). Practical recommendations are to limit assumptions made by treating clinicians that patients will agree to a gynaecological examination at the first visit. Efforts to be made by the specialist to keep contact with the patient by sitting on the same level and offering space for a support person to be in the room are suggested. Furthermore, choosing one's language carefully is important. Referring to an 'examination table' rather than 'bed' is considered important. While the patient might complete informed consent to be examined, if there is any difficulty with using a speculum or swab, this can be taken as a sign to pause, to enquire about the client's well-being and to adjust the plan of care (Owens et al., 2001, p. 4). Asking the client what parts of the consultation or procedure are likely to be triggering should be part of the consultation. Giving the client the power to stop the examination process whenever they feel uncomfortable is recommended. If the survivor agrees to be examined, practical steps such as keeping the patient well covered by draping the patient's body with blankets, watching for signs of hyperarousal/anxiety and expressing a willingness to postpone examination are proposed. Giving the client privacy after the examination to get dressed and debriefing by asking the client what went well and what could be improved upon are suggested. This evaluation can then inform future consultations if examinations are needed regularly (Owens et al., 2021, p. 4).

Pregnancy checks, giving birth and aftercare involve a number of potentially triggering interventions that require careful attention from clinicians who are dealing with women who are survivors of CSA. Having a current pregnancy requires ongoing examinations and scans that are potentially triggering of issues related to CSA. As the case study of Lisa in Chapter Two illustrated, abuse issues can be recollected at any time during a pregnancy or during intrusive fertility treatments. This can impact a decision to try again after conception or pregnancy fails. Flashpoints of distress are common throughout the pregnancy journey, as the case study of Roz illustrates.

Case study 3: Roz

Roz is a 32-year-old Australian-born woman who has news of a long-awaited first pregnancy. At three months into the pregnancy, she began having depressive symptoms, which she had experienced earlier in her life.

Roz had difficulties her father with whom she had an anxious-ambivalent attachment due to his coming and going in and out of a relationship with her mother. As an adult, she learned that he had a diagnosis of bipolar affective disorder that was kept secret from her. His mental health condition was considered a source of shame within his family, and this had been felt by her mother, who was stigmatised by her family of origin with which there was little contact. As Roz's father was often an inconsistent figure on whom she could not rely, she felt him to be untrustworthy. She been a victim of sexual abuse at his hands when she stayed with him during school holidays. He would involve her in 'games' that provided opportunities for him to molest her by touching her intimately through her clothing. She was only nine years old at the time, and, though she tried to tell her mother, these accounts were dismissed and ignored as being part of his bipolar affective disorder. To keep herself safe, she decided she would stop staying with her father during school holidays.

Roz said these feelings related to her CSA and not being believed were reignited by the bodily feeling of being pregnant. She had been unwell with hyperemesis, a persistent cycle of nausea commonly caused by hormonal changes during pregnancy. She mentioned her worries about the developing baby not getting all the sustenance it needed from her owing to her vomiting and difficulty eating and drinking. This conversation was attempted with her doctor, who reassured her that 'the foetus would take what it needed' via the placenta. Ever since this comment, Roz had a vision of carrying a parasite that was drawing on her bodily reserves, which were depleted by the hyperemesis. She had experienced morning sickness during the early weeks of the pregnancy to the extent that she was unable to keep down any solid food and, at times, even water. This miserable time had rekindled the sense of being out of control. Roz felt the medical professionals minimised her distress, and this raised past feelings of being disbelieved and betrayed by her mother when she was a child. She had expected her first pregnancy to be a happy and contented time but she rapidly became unwell. She felt vulnerable as she could not work owing to the constant nausea.

Fortunately, the obstetrician had some knowledge of trauma-informed care and had referred Roz to the hospital social worker for follow-up. Within that context, Roz was able to retell her story of the CSA and how it had impacted her life. With trauma-informed, supportive contact, the social worker facilitated a revised birth plan so that Roz began to feel more in control over her delivery. As her new anti-nausea medication helped with her symptoms, she returned to work and planned to work from home more, in a familiar environment where she would be able to rest if necessary.

Roz was referred to see me when her baby daughter was three months old, a healthy and well-adjusted baby. Roz was having difficulty sleeping. Roz told me that she had worries about her baby dying while she was asleep. When I connected with her, she was exhausted, and so we looked at options for respite care so that she would have some rest time during the day while her baby was taken care of. Roz feared leaving her baby in the care of a professional child carer, and so that option was not acceptable to her. She told me of her CSA to contextualise why she felt compelled to protect her baby, to give her daughter a better experience of parenting than she had had. The pressure to be a better parent than her own parents seemed to be at the heart of her concerns, which were compounding her anxiety and leading to the insomnia. It was as though she feared that her child would be taken away from her and this was out of her control. We explored ways that she could feel more in control of her life, and she came up with a plan that helped her anxiety and insomnia that involved her partner taking time off from his work to care for the baby at night, as he was aware of Roz's CSA and the impact on her as an adult. This revised plan, going forward, seemed to be working for Roz, whose general health and well-being improved in the weeks following.

Further reflections on the case studies of Roz and Kayla

Considering every woman seen in women's health as a potential trauma survivor would be a paradigm shift assisting health professionals to develop a heightened respect of survivors of CSA. In a wider sense, an approach that shares power would also benefit all women patients. Articles such as the one written by medical specialists and researchers would assist in the sharing of practical tips for safely performing medical examinations. Rather than seeking details of women survivors' abuse, clinicians need to power share in order to produce a co-created dialogue with survivors when dealing with reproductive and other forms of women's health care, particularly when intrusive procedures are required (Owens et al., 2021).

In the case study, Roz's original abuse narrative was triggered by the physical changes her body was undergoing during pregnancy. This is a relatively common response and is a time when CSA can arise. In reliving her CSA, she was considering how to be a better parent compared to the caregiving she experienced in her family of origin. The difficulties Roz had with her pregnancy were a response to her need to revisit the impact of her

CSA in order to get through her pregnancy and birth experience and begin the parenting of her daughter. With the help of her supportive partner and medical and social work team, she managed her traumatic past that was reignited by the pregnancy, birth and parenting challenges.

Kayla

The education goals that Kayla had for her life in the first case study had been challenged by her decision to end an exploitative relationship. Her past abuse had meant that her parents had been very protective of her since the time when she had disclosed her CSA as a 12 year old. Kayla wanted to avoid their input, however, as she was trying to make an independent adult decision about her life. The potential for shame is a common response to CSA. As she did not initially reach out to others having withdrawn socially, she manifested her psychological pain in thoughts of self-harm and suicidality.

Kayla had a wish to become a parent. Her life goal of becoming a mother seemed out of reach because of a recurring pattern of getting into abusive relationships and then realising she needed to leave the partner. Her vision for her future life included a two-person family where she felt loved and supported. This quality of intimate relationship she was desperate to have seemed to her to be unavailable in her past and current relationships, triggering despair, grief and feelings of abandonment. Kayla felt she would never be able to realise her dreams for the future. Through exploring her inner critic and increasing her capacity to reach out to others, she could once again see a semblance of a future.

Conclusion

Health care providers need trauma-informed theory and care to be an integrated part of their professional training and ongoing professional development. It is of critical importance to understand what helps and what hinders the disclosure process for women survivors of CSA as women take on adult life roles in partnerships, education, careers and parenting. Educating significant others, who might include non-family members such as friends and partners, about responding appropriately to the woman needs to be an integral part of the care offered by all helping professionals. A holistic focus on the well-being of the woman within extended family and friend networks, culture and gender beliefs is, therefore, recommended. As women are seen as responsible for keeping the family together, they may worry about disclosing their historical abuse within their family of origin for fear of breaking the family up. Therefore, gender and culture can be both facilitators and barriers to disclosure. For helping professionals, this forms a valuable knowledge base from which to learn and practise.

Some confidents to whom survivors disclose may face challenges managing their emotional reactions in order to fully hear and comprehend what is told to them. Planning for and rehearsing a retrospective disclosure of CSA is a useful part of the preparation for the range of responses that women survivors of CSA might receive in the retelling. Encouraging sensitivity to what might be a safe environment for disclosure may be usefully explored. If the first attempt at disclosure is not met positively or elicits a reaction of anger from others, withdrawal, pity or other responses found to be harmful, processing this response can provide a springboard for the survivor to avoid going down the 'shame spiral'. Fostering hope that there may be a more positive response from others in time, if a negative response has been experienced, is also important.

In the next chapter, the midlife phase is explored for women survivors of CSA. Here, the challenges of empty nest syndrome, with children leaving home, can bring matters from earlier in life into sharp relief. Partnerships that have offered a lifelong witness to the effects of CSA may be challenged for various reasons, creating a choice point for revision, change and consolidation for the future.

References

Alaggia, R. (2005). Disclosing the trauma of child sexual abuse: a gender analysis. *Journal of Trauma and Loss*, 10(5), 453–470.

Alaggia, R., Collin-Vezina, D., & Lateef, R. (2019). Facilitators and barriers to child sexual abuse (CSA) disclosures: a research update (2000–2016). *Trauma, Violence, and Abuse*, 20(2), 260–283. doi:10.1177/1524838017697312

Bolen, R. M., & Lamb, J. L. (2004). Ambivalence of nonoffending guardians after child sexual abuse disclosure. *Journal of Interpersonal Violence*, 19(2), 185–211. doi:10.1177/0886260503260324

De Montigny Gauthier, L., Vaillancourt-Morel, M. P., Rellini, A., Godbout, N., Charbonneau-Lefebvre, V., Desjardins, F., & Bergeron, S. (2019). The risk of telling: a dyadic perspective on romantic partners' responses to child sexual abuse disclosure and their associations with sexual and relationship satisfaction. *Journal of Marital and Family Therapy*, 45(3), 480–493.

Epston, D., & White, M. (1992). *Experience, Contradiction, Narrative & Imagination: Selected Papers of David Epston & Michael White, 1989–1991*. Dulwich Centre.

Guyon, R., Fernet, M., Dussault, E., Gauthier-Duchesne, A., Cousineau, M. M., Tardif, M., & Godbout, N. (2021). Experiences of disclosure and reactions of close ones from the perspective of child sexual abuse survivors: a qualitative analysis of gender specificities. *Journal of Child Sexual Abuse*, 30(7), 806–827. doi:10.1080/10538712.2021.1942369

Halvorsen, J. E., Solberg, E. T., & Stige, S. H. (2020). "To say it out loud is to kill your own childhood." – An exploration of the first person perspective of barriers to disclosing child sexual abuse. *Children and Youth Services Review*, 113. doi:10.1016/j.childyouth.2020.104999

Hatuqa, D. (2018). Muslim women chart their own path in #MeToo era. GlobalPost. Retrieved 17 August 2024 from https://theworld.org/stories/2018/12/20/muslim-women-chart-their-own-path-metoo-era

Herman, J. (1992). *Trauma and Recovery*. Basic Books.

Herman, J. (2015). *Trauma and Recovery*. Basic Books.

MacGinley, M., Breckenridge, J., & Mowll, J. (2019). A scoping review of adult survivors' experiences of shame following sexual abuse in childhood. *Health and Social Care in the Community*, 27(5), 1135–1146. doi:10.1111/hsc.12771

Owens, L., Terrell, S., Low, L. K., Loder, C., Rhizal, D., Scheiman, L., & Seng, J. (2021). Universal precautions: the case for consistently trauma-informed reproductive healthcare. *American Journal of Obstetrics and Gynecology*, 226(5), 671–677. doi:10.1016/j.ajog.2021.08.012

Stige, S. H., Halvorsen, J. E., & Solberg, E. T. (2020). Pathways to understanding – how adult survivors of child sexual abuse came to understand that they had been sexually abused. *Journal of Child Sexual Abuse*, 29(2), 205–221.

Tener, D., & Murphy, S. B. (2015). Adult disclosure of child sexual abuse: a literature review. *Trauma Violence Abuse*, 16(4), 391–400. doi:10.1177/1524838014537906

Wallis, C. R. D., & Woodworth, M. (2021). Non-offending caregiver support in cases of child sexual abuse: an examination of the impact of support on formal disclosures. *Child Abuse and Neglect*, 113. doi:10.1016/j.chiabu.2021.104929

White, M. (1995). *Re-authoring Lives: Interviews and Essays.* Dulwich Centre.

World Health Organization (WHO). (2017). Guidelines on sexual abuse of children. Retrieved 11 November from www.who.int/violence injury prevention/resources/publications/en/guidelines

5 Midlife – change, consolidation, reformulated identity and the way forward

Midlife – change, consolidation, the past and the way forward

> The joint meetings enabled us to realise how important we were to each other. … It showed us that the new unit we were creating posed an opportunity for a corrective emotional experience and embodied hope.
>
> (Adult survivor of CSA reflecting on her couple therapy undertaken in an attempt to free her relationship with her partner from the impact of historical CSA; Nasim & Nadan, 2013, p. 375)

Introduction

In this chapter, we explore the disclosure of CSA by women in the middle years of life (40–60). This phase of the lifespan can be a time of change, diversification and the consolidation of work, family commitments and the growth of one's personal identity. Most women experience menopause at some point during this period, spelling the end of their fertile years and reproductive potential with the experience of perimenopause and menopause. Relationships can alter in midlife as a consequence of changing priorities or empty nest syndrome with children leaving home, freeing up more time for career development and the pursuit of other life goals amid revised aspirations. For many women, it is a time when careers are reviewed with a view to changing direction or finding more fulfilment in different areas of life.

As illustrated in Chapter Two with the case study of Lisa and her husband, John, if women survivors have focused on paid work throughout their adult lives, the wish to have a child may become more prominent and attempts may be made to conceive a first pregnancy after the age of 40. Having children in midlife can involve a change of lifestyle as well as the notion of a career encompassing the new role of becoming a parent. For other women, who have had their children earlier, in their teens and 20s, by this age, they may face a crisis caused by adolescent children seeking greater independence, leaving home to attend university or to live with peers, focusing on the development their own adult relationships. Some are faced with the prospect of welcoming the next generation by becoming grandparents. When faced by such major change and milestones, there can be a sense of needing to reinvent

DOI: 10.4324/9781032669205-5

oneself after years of parenting in order to mark the shift to another phase of life, with a revised sense of self and identity.

The partial disclosure of CSA by women in their teens, 20s and 30s can be revisited in midlife with an enhanced sense of personal agency and power in this phase due to the accumulated experiential knowledge gained in the previous decades of life. This increased awareness can be about oneself and the contexts of one's life, and about the world more generally. Sometimes, there can be a desire for formal disclosure of CSA to authorities as the survivor may have integrated survivorship into her identity and now seeks redress for what happened in the past as a way of planning for the future. Psychological healing can again become prominent, and financial compensation may be sought as a symbol of transforming the past into an acknowledgement that the abuse happened and affected her life. Seeking formal acknowledgement of and redress for grievances relating to the abuse and connected family relationships can be important in this phase of life as another attempt is made at disclosure in the hope of putting the past in its place once and for all.

The disclosure process – from adolescence to middle age

To recap previous chapters, in a review of how disclosure of CSA can proceed, most children and adolescents were discovered to delay telling anyone about their abuse until adulthood (McElvaney, 2015).The delay in disclosure can be for up to 49 years according to one research review, with an average delay in making disclosure of CSA of 21 years (Jonson & Lindblad, 2004, cited in McElvaney, 2015, p. 161). Those who disclosed as adolescents most often told only one close confident, who was usually a peer or friend of similar age (Jonson & Lindblad, 2004, cited in McElvaney, 2015, p. 161). The evidence base on the obstacles and facilitators of disclosure has led to an acknowledgement of the importance of peer relationships in the disclosure of CSA. Involving school friends in the disclosure process brings a sense of safety to many adolescent women survivors, as they may fear the consequences of disclosing to parents. Peers, rather than parents, as the first witnesses and responders to disclosure are emphasised in the literature on disclosure of CSA by women. Direct questioning of something being wrong by other significant others beyond family can also prompt the disclosure of CSA (McElvaney et al., 2014). Finding ways of assessing safety in the peer relationship for facilitating this disclosure is thought to involve an ongoing assessment of trustworthiness until the peer is thought to be a trustworthy confident. How, with the survivor's consent, the peer is able to bring these disclosures to the attention of responsible adults, for professional or family support, is an area for further research and development. Learning how to bridge the divide between the disclosure to peers and moving disclosure to the responsible adult in the woman's life has critical practice implications for the adult woman survivor's healing journey. If the peer does not go at the woman's pace and respect the need for confidentiality, he or she may lose the confidence of the survivor who has disclosed to them.

McElvaney's (2015) theorising about the disclosure process for survivors of CSA aligns with other research findings about the facilitators of and barriers to CSA disclosure. As summarised in the preceding chapters, the fear of the consequences of disclosing CSA during childhood is still being identified as a predictor of delayed disclosure (McElvaney, 2015, p. 163). Older children are more likely to disclose than younger children as they are able to draw from their internalised sense of whether they will be believed and have the competence to judge/estimate the consequences of telling others (McElvaney, 2015).

Wager (2013), in reviewing the studies on disclosure of CSA, concludes that most adults experience periods of unawareness of their CSA before fully realising what has happened to them in childhood. This unawareness of CSA may be hypothesised to be a survival strategy that enables a child who is dependent on her caregiver to continue to engage in their usual behaviours to elicit the care they need at this stage in development. The tendency towards amnesia or dissociation is more prevalent when the abuser is a parent than when it is someone from outside the child's family according to other studies, including those conducted over a number of years (Wager, 2013, p. 883). A negative response to disclosure by responsible adults in the child's life increases the potential for the child or young person to develop dissociation and amnesia, which can delay the disclosure until much later in life. This amnesia or dissociation is found to be prominent when the perpetrator is a primary caregiver. In these circumstances, the child or young person may more often internalise what is happening as being their fault, or the act of disclosure is framed as being 'bad' by the recipient of the disclosure. Through the dynamic of shame, the child is imbued with a sense of 'badness' attributed by the act of disclosure to the person who negatively responds to the disclosure (Wager, 2013). Furthermore, if the child is abused in childhood by a close family member and internalises the responsibility to herself, she is more likely to be abused subsequently in adolescence (Wager, 2013). If the abuse is disclosed in childhood, the author discovered, from reviewing the evidence-based literature, that the child may be at risk of further sexual or physical abuse by the disbelieving family member (Wager, 2013).

The pervasive nature of shame as a barrier to disclosure

The shame/self-stigmatisation cycle outlined in Chapter Four can be a continuing barrier to making any disclosure, including in midlife, when the survivor comes to see the actions of her childhood self through adult eyes. Recognition of her CSA can, for example, be reflected on as a middle-aged woman seeing her risk-taking actions as an adolescent as representing a cry for help. Self-blame and an internalised sense of shame are promoted by the continuing disbelief or blaming by the person disclosed to. Most often, a mother or mother-type figure is disclosed to. Such disclosures to a responsible adult are conceptualised as a 'double betrayal', perpetuating dissociation and highlighting the identity-tarnishing effect of the disclosure when the disclosure is disbelieved. Disclosure of CSA runs the risk of incurring the wrath of the confident (Wager, 2013). This refocusing of attention from the survivor's internalised sense of shame and stigmatisation enables the perpetrator's actions to be seen more clearly as opportunistically or planned exploitation of the child's vulnerability. The various ways in which the perpetrator reframed the abuse as 'evidence of specialness', 'game playing' or 'experimentation with sex' can now be viewed as being part of the process of 'grooming' the vulnerable child or adolescent for sexual abuse.

For all these reasons, therefore, disclosure might be delayed until middle age, when a woman may feel more confident and entitled to initially disclose or to try telling again. She may have tackled 'the double betrayal' of having had a negative response to disclosure from the non-abusing parent or guardian by this stage in life. This stepping out of the shame spiral, described in Chapter Four, is described for survivors with increasing age, as we will also see highlighted in the next chapter when discussing the experiences of women survivors in the 60+ age range. From the middle years onwards, matured insights about one's life increasingly become available, and some things are seen with greater clarity than previously. Seeing the perpetrator as being the person at fault is a feature of detaching from the shame/self-stigmatising cycle, which survivors can be engaged in for much of life. This detachment from the self-stigmatising process can be helpful in presenting possibilities for retelling, including exploration of the options for reporting the abuse to the authorities. Searching for an alternative means of obtaining justice may involve seeking compensation in various ways, such as volunteering for public inquiries, royal commissions on abuse in institutional care, and returning to family to attempt to obtain redress for their CSA.

Witnessing opportunities for initial disclosure and re-disclosure

When a formal public investigation into CSA occurs, prompted by growing public awareness of the need for policy change, such as during government-commissioned inquiries, opportunities can emerge for formal disclosure many years after the CSA. A recent example involving survivors of CSA was the royal commission in New Zealand involving abuse within institutional care. The Australian inquiry into abuse in the church or religious domain is yet another example of public recognition of the impact of transgressed boundaries and of CSA throughout life. This kind of public inquiry can signal to women survivors of CSA the need to revisit the past as royal commissions provide an independent investigation and further opportunity to come forward to disclose childhood sexual abuse in these contexts. Investigations into institutions such as the church, child protection services, schools, university halls of residence and sporting associations where survivors have been sexually abused are other examples of contexts where survivors are able to tell their stories, which are recorded and heard and reheard, leading to various forms of redress for the grievance expressed. Remedies ranging from financial compensation to therapy, recommendations for policy and institutional change, and mediation are often offered as an outcome of such public inquiries.

The couple context as a 'liminal space'

Where there is a partner who has been with the woman survivor for the duration of her adult life, there can be a witnessing of the woman's journey of healing from CSA within the partnership over time. Nasim and Nadan (2013) propose a model of couple counselling that they refer to as 'twofold witnessing' in which the therapist witnesses how the past CSA has or is affecting the dynamics of the couple relationship, while the partner of the woman witnesses her own healing from CSA as an adult (Nasim & Nadan, 2013). As the fragments of memory of CSA can be experienced as sensory recollections, they can reoccur as states of consciousness that are beyond conscious thought and may be expressed in the intimacy of the couple relationship through patterns discerned in close relationships. These interactions can be various re-enactments of the original abuse. Consequently, the couple relationship can become the crucible for healing from CSA from Nasim and Nadan's perspective (2013, p. 370).

Added to this theorising, the act of witnessing occurs in what I have conceptualised elsewhere as a 'liminal space', which is a holding space between the old way of life and the new (Pack, 2009). As we have seen in the previous chapters, through attachment and interaction within protective and nurturing relationships, the woman survivor of CSA is enabled to reconnect the fragments of memory of her CSA. The buffering or protective factors ameliorating the shame and self-blame that lead to dissociation and isolation come from the social connection within the trusting relationship. These protective factors coalesce through the security of the adult attachment, providing an environment in which to both initiate and continue the disclosure process.

The New Trauma therapists, such as Herman (1992), advocate the healing potential of a relationship or connection in which the supporter witnesses the effects of the CSA. This witnessing has the potential to transform the original CSA through the survivor feeling able to attach new meaning to experience when in relationship to a trusted other. The context of a relationship of trust with a helping professional such as a therapist provides the safe container in which issues related to CSA and their effects can be explored. Adult intimate relationships with friends and partners further this potential for healing from CSA, depending on the perceived trustworthiness of the partner in the survivor's eyes and on the quality of this relationship.

In the act of witnessing, Herman specifically refers to the therapists' attending to the injustice of the CSA, with therapy seen as being a social justice as well as individual intervention (Herman, 1992). In the couple context, the partner witnesses the broader biography of the survivor and the impacts on their life together. In Nasim and Nadan's (2013) model, the therapist enters the dynamics of the couple relationship to witness traumatic relationship patterns so that these can be named and transformed through their identification. In relation to the couple, the couple counsellor aims to identify patterns of interaction using Michael White's theorising within the framework for narrative therapy he developed with clients who became enmeshed in 'problem-saturated' narratives. Some of the cases discussed related to abuse survivors who were operating from these 'problem-saturated' narratives that led to their living limited lives with a loss of hope for their future. The concept of 'externalising the problem' is emphasised, where the problems of relating as a couple are reframed as being fleeting patterns of interaction rather than being intractable and belonging to either person in the relationship (White, 1995).

White's theory development in narrative therapy in turn draws from the work of Barbara Myerhoff, a cultural anthropologist who, influenced by the work of Turner (1969), developed the notion of 'liminal space' (Myerhoff, 1982). As outlined in previous chapters, Myerhoff conceptualised this reflective process of remembering and connection of past trauma within present safety as occurring in a 'liminal space', a transitional zone (Myerhoff, 1982). I have conceptualised 'liminal space' in terms of the healing from sexual abuse trauma as the survivor, in her therapy, finds the language for speaking the unspeakable. In this process of remembering, from disclosure to managing the ongoing aftermath of disclosure and the effects of CSA, she exists with the person confided in, in a liminal space of new meaning making. It is a conceptual holding space, a place of betwixt and between, akin to the departure lounge at the airport where the new destination can be imagined from the familiarity of the known world (Pack, 2002; Pack, 2013).

In Nasim and Nadan's (2013) study, they propose that, once the survivor has established the position of the partner, who is coached to listen as a detached bystander, they enter a place akin to a liminal space. The survivor is encouraged to tell her story of how the abuse impacts her life as the partner listens and witnesses her account. When the survivor has completed her narrative, the partner is permitted to respond, reflecting on what they learned. This background assists the partner to better understand the triggers in their relating that evoke issues from the past abuse for the woman survivor of CSA. Prompts are given by the therapist to the partner to open up a dialogue between the woman who has told her story and the outsider (the partner) who listens to it. Once this safe context is established, the scene is set for other conversations about problems with different aspects of the relationship and how the origins of many are related to the legacy of coping with CSA over many decades (Nasim & Nadan, 2013, p. 375).

When the woman survivor has a lifelong partner who has witnessed her healing journey over time, there can be challenges in navigating normal life transitions, such as empty nest syndrome, health crises, restructuring at work/redundancy, planning for retirement and looking towards later lives together with grandchildren. The following case study explores one example of a 55-year-old receptionist whose two daughters were both about to leave home to attend university. Her husband then faced a cancer diagnosis that threatened his career, their financial security and their future plans for retirement. In couple counselling with Rob, she chose to begin her narrative in adolescence when she first met her husband-to-be. Their relationship provided a 'liminal space' in which she was able to find healing from CSA through the quality of trust in her relationship with him.

Risk and protective factors in the case of Shelia

Shelia had a troubled adolescence. When she was 13, her mother, Betty, stopped her going out socially and had rigid rules in place at home that were a source of conflict between mother and daughter. Her birth father had abruptly left home after an argument when Shelia was five years old. Her uncle (her mother's brother), Tom, then came to live with them and stayed living with them until Shelia was eight years old. He took on a parental role within the household to help his sister parent Shelia. Shelia, as an adult, recalls some inappropriate behaviour with Tom when she was a child, as he often would walk around the house in the nude and expose himself to Shelia. She felt, as an adult, that his contact with her was sexualised and inappropriate, although she didn't identify the 'yukky feelings' until now. As a child, she told her mother about Tom's conduct when she went out to work and they were alone in the house, but Betty said Shelia was 'making it up' because she missed her father and craved more of her mother's attention to compensate. When Shelia told the class about her uncle during morning talk with her classmates, the teacher present was deeply troubled by the child's story and decided to report her Uncle Tom's conduct to the authorities. A child protection social worker visited Shelia and her mother to investigate Shelia's safety. Her mother denied any inappropriate conduct and told the social worker that her brother, Tom, had moved out of the house now, which he did shortly after this visit, and that she did not know where he had gone subsequently.

Shelia ran away from home continually after this owing to the double betrayal of the sexualised conduct of her maternal uncle and her mother's denial of what had happened with him. Shelia felt there was no one to protect her from the inappropriateness of male relatives and she did not wish to have contact with her uncle after that. She found school and her relationships with peers and teachers to be a stabilising influence at this time, as she felt safe with her friends at school and with the teachers who were aware of the difficulties at home. Because of what was happening at home, Shelia often missed classes and truanted with her best friend at a local shopping mall, with her mother being unaware of the lack of school attendance. This brought Shelia to the attention of the child protection services again, who became involved owing to the school's concerns about the absences from class. The social worker could see that Shelia's mother was struggling as a single parent to cope with Shelia's acting out with her and truanting behaviour. It seemed as though mother and daughter were engaged in a battle of wills, with Shelia running away when she felt her mother was not listening to what she was saying. The child protection social worker organised for Shelia to go into respite foster care with a family who had an adolescent daughter, in the hope that this would assist the mother's and daughter's relationship and with the truanting issue at school.

As Shelia had a good friend at school with whose family she often stayed, it was to her girlfriend and her family that she felt safe to confide about what happened in that foster placement. Shelia took being moved into placement with a foster family, albeit temporarily, as bringing with it a sense of her own power after the unwillingness of her mother to believe and so protect her. She concluded that no adult could manage her behaviour and so she felt she could challenge her foster carers also. This led to changes of foster care placement as the families found her too rebellious to parent. Owing to the constant change of foster carers, she also had a sense of nobody wanting her and an internalised sense of something being wrong with her. She told her social worker she would be 'better next time'.

Within one of her foster care families, there was an older son, aged 16 years, who sexually abused Shelia while his parents (the foster carers) were engaged with their other children, who were much younger. Shelia was 14 years at the time. She never told the authorities as she thought this was something she needed to put up with or she would be returned home to her mother. The abuse consisted of her foster brother visiting her after school in her bedroom, where she was raped whenever the foster parents were not in the vicinity. Shelia disclosed what was happening to her girlfriend, who kept her confidentiality about the abuse as Shelia felt the shame of what was happening and had internalised it as being, in some way, her own fault. She felt she was deserving of the punishment for rebelling against her mother and knew her mother wouldn't believe her if she told her.

Shelia asked the child protection social worker for a change of placement, but none was available, and so she remained in that situation for a year. Eventually, at age 15 years, she moved to stay with her girlfriend's family. It was in closely confiding in her school friend in the position of relative safety that she disclosed the sexual abuse to her friend's parents. They then informed the child protection social worker involved in her care.

Risk and protective factors in the case of Shelia

Being at school, with the continuity of her peer group, was the major protective factor for Shelia as she was growing up after her abuse during her teens. It was around this time that she met her future partner, Rob, who was her boyfriend as a 16 year old and a year ahead of her at the same college. They were high school sweethearts until they left school for their big overseas travel experience in their later teens, with Rob returning with her to introduce her to his extended family in Scotland. Staying with his extended family provided her with an alternative experience of family, which was experienced by Shelia as being warmly welcoming and supportive. Rob and Shelia had a working holiday in the UK to enable them to travel as backpackers to many European countries; then, after three years, they returned to New Zealand to marry, find jobs and establish a home together. Time away from New Zealand in overseas destinations freed Shelia from traumatic memories of the past, which she had found to be extraordinarily liberating. Being supported by Rob and his family was challenging to begin with but became familiar, and her sense of safety with them increased.

Shelia did suffer periods of dissociation where she would appear to be present but, emotionally, she seemed too remote to others. At these times, she would want to isolate. She realised that she used to do this with her peers at high school, including Rob, as a way of regaining the control she felt she had lost during her abuse in foster care. As her relationship with Rob developed and deepened, and they had their two daughters, she felt the sadness of dissociating, which meant that she withdrew emotionally. Because of this, she saw that he could not know some aspects about her. She wanted him to understand this coping mechanism but was afraid that he would leave and abandon her if she talked openly about this.

In his 40s, Rob developed a form of blood cancer, the diagnosis of which came as a huge shock to Shelia, who relied on Rob to be 'her rock'. She now faced the prospect of being in a caregiver's role during his chemotherapy. When his treatment was completed, she noticed herself becoming angry with him, commenting: 'what am I meant to do if you die? I can't find someone again because of everything that has happened in my life'. With this comment, she realised that she was assuming that all cancer diagnoses end in death, and that this prospect raised the spectre of early abandonment by her primary caregiver, her mother, with the descent into foster care where she was abused.

In couple therapy, they were able to speak individually about the impact of Shelia's abuse on their relationship. Rob was mindful to let Shelia have time on her own when she was feeling dissociated and recognised the non-verbal indicators that she was physically there but not actually emotionally present at some points in time, particularly when under stress. He had learned to see these times as important to Shelia and recognised a need to be respectful by allowing her time and space to recover.

When he told Shelia what he had noticed of her process, she hadn't realised that he knew about her dissociation, which she said she had tried to keep secret from all the family. Rob said he didn't like to think that he was causing any distress for Shelia, particularly during intimate contact, and so he often felt he needed to 'back off' too at these times. On hearing Rob talk about this, she was moved by his sensitivity to her needs and asked him not to back off but to ask what was wrong and to listen, as she needed to talk at those times rather than to isolate herself. Rob was keen to try this enquiring, when he noticed her withdrawing, between sessions.

At the next session, the therapist encouraged Rob to ask any questions he might have about other responses he found confusing. He mentioned that he wanted to understand Shelia's worries and concerns and would silently listen in a non-judgemental way. Through the therapist establishing a context for witnessing, Shelia was able to tell and retell the story of her abuse and how it had transformed her life. She realised in that witnessing of her own narrative that she did not want to be without the support of Rob with whom her life story continued to be transformed from victimhood into survivorship. The daily happy experience of their lives, together with their two daughters, who were now reaching the stage of leaving home, was central to Shelia's well-being. Shelia realised her daughters were about the same age as she was when she was abused in foster care and so she recognised the re-enactment of themes from her earlier life through observing their growing independence from her.

Reflection on the case study of Shelia

As mentioned in Chapter Four, women survivors of CSA often turn to their peers when relationships with adults lack the psychological safety within which to disclose the abuse they have experienced. Shelia disclosed her abuse to her best friend, and the friend's parents then reported her abuse to the child protection authorities with Shelia's consent. This peer support and adoptive family support mirrors some of the findings of Chapters Three and Four where one of the main protective factors enabling disclosure involves a quality of unconditional positive regard of significant others who believe and support the teen or childhood survivor of sexual abuse.

The second main protective factor in Shelia's upbringing was the lifelong relationship with her first boyfriend, forged in her teens, that developed into being a lifelong partnership. Her childhood sweetheart turned into her future partner, Rob. By establishing a network of relationships around her, Shelia had the protective factors of the school and friend networks surrounding her in which it felt safe enough to disclose to her boyfriend, who was her first consensual sexual partner. The manifold after-effects of CSA were revisited by Shelia under the caring gaze of her husband throughout their marriage.

Her life partnership provided her with confidence and opportunities to move outside her country of origin to work and travel overseas in her late teens and 20s, by which she was able to leave behind some of the negative memories of her upbringing and the past. While on a working holiday in the UK with her future husband, she was introduced to a new culture and became part of a new family, with her in-laws providing a new perspective of what belonging to a family and clan in Scotland was like. In the warmth of these new relationships she married, returned to her country of origin and established a new identity as a married woman who became a medical receptionist, with a stable home life, and, in the fullness of time, started a family.

Rob's health crisis provided a challenge to the lifelong witnessing he had of Shelia's early schooling and teenage years, their travels together, their commitment to supporting one another, experiences of parenting and, ultimately, their life together. In couple therapy, they took turns to notice how the past abuse impacted their relationship, encouraging each other to take responsibility for holding back from entering re-enactments based in the past. Shelia was able to say she was afraid of losing Rob during his treatment for cancer, and Rob was able to hear this rather than her outrage and anger at feeling abandoned as she had felt by her mother, which had led to the foster care arrangement. Shelia felt supported to tell Rob who her abuser was, as he was known to Rob. Rob wanted to understand why Shelia had left it so long to tell him this and asked how long the abuse went on for. He wanted to know if there was anything he did that triggered Shelia into remembering her abuse at times when she seemed remote. She mentioned she always disliked him seeing her in the shower when he was in the bathroom as it reminded her of being observed in the shower by her perpetrator before he raped her in her bedroom. Rob wept when he heard this as he had no idea and was so sad to hear that Shelia had to endure such indignities. His anger towards the perpetrator led to his having some individual sessions with another therapist as their couple work continued.

For Shelia, she struggled with the shame that is often a pervasive and lingering aftermath of CSA. Her individual therapy worked well for her, and she was able to begin to see the problems in adulthood more as the aftermath of the shame she experienced in adolescence. She now put the blame for the abuse back with the perpetrator and, through her protective attitudes towards her teenage daughters, could have greater compassion for herself during her childhood and teen years. The feelings of abandonment by her mother were also part of the context of her CSA, and so it was important in her healing to reflect on her style of parenting her daughters, which, in some ways, she was able to see was part of a legacy of her own abuse and experiences as a child and young person.

Rob is still in remission from cancer, and, while he is on medication still, their life together continues now, with both their daughters living in university halls and studying towards degrees.

Protective and risk factors in the case of Shelia

Shelia had the protective factor of positive peer relationships and academic and social functioning at school, which was a significant buffer against feeling unworthy, and so she tended not to hide, self-isolate or cut herself off from others in her peer group. Although she had an ambivalent-avoidant attachment style and ongoing conflictual relationship with her mother, she was able to develop trust in peer relationships. Her teacher had assessed her disclosure of abuse without Shelia being aware of the import of what she had said and how it would be seen by others. Through the involvement of the child protection services, her home life changed, although, because of the running away from home, she was placed in foster care. Previous research has found that young women who have a pattern of running away from home have a sexual risk trajectory of being sexually abused again in the year after their running away (Thrane et al, 2011). Neglect from the primary caregiver that continues after running away behaviour is thought to predispose adolescent women to an increased risk of subsequent sexual assault. In Shelia's foster care placements, there had been aspects of neglect by her foster parents as well as neglect from her own mother.

Within her peer relationships, she was fortunate to form an intimate relationship with her boyfriend, who grew to be her life partner. Their respective work and parenting roles occurred in the context of a loving and supportive relationship that assisted Shelia's recovery from CSA.

After the couple counselling sessions

While there were some aspects of their life that continued to be impacted by the effects of CSA, as a couple Shelia and Rob were working out what these aspects were and finding a way of moving forward so that these did not impair their lives together as a couple. Shelia came forward to tell her story of abuse when there was a royal inquiry into abuse in institutional care, established in New Zealand in 2022. This inquiry has been investigating why people entered state care in the first place, what experiences of abuse they reported and the ongoing effects of this abuse on the individual survivor and her *whānau*/wider community (Royal Commission of Inquiry, 2024).

By late 2022, over 2,700 survivors of CSA (and other forms of abuse that occurred in state care) had come forward to be interviewed to provide evidence for the inquiry. The aim of gathering the survivor narratives is to examine these accounts alongside the responses of state agencies explaining their role in the abuse and neglect of young people and vulnerable adults during public hearings.

Shelia said her motivation for giving evidence at this point in her life was to ensure that changes were made so that that the factors that allowed for her sexual abuse to occur in the past do not continue today and into the future. She wanted to make a difference to the lives of other young people who became disconnected from their parents and then went on to be in foster care. The final report of the inquiry has yet to be published, but, at the time of writing, the inquiry has said that: 'we cannot make any findings, reach any conclusions or make recommendations without hearing the voices of those who have the lived experience of state or faith based care' (Royal Commission of Inquiry, 2024).

The implications for practice

Gaining a greater awareness of the shame/self-stigmatisation spiral can assist survivors to break out of the self-imposed silence that often surrounds the abuse and keeps the effects ongoing in their lives. When they realise they can make a difference, in their individual lives and by choosing to tell their stories of survival through such inquiries, a sense of unworthiness can be transformed into becoming a self-advocate and an agent of social change in society. Most children interviewed by McElvaney et al. (2014) found that young persons' disclosure of CSA was prompted in two ways. The first was the 'pressure cooker' effect of shoring up strong emotions that manifested in two main ways. One was internal to the individual survivor, who began to act in a way that was out of character, and this change in behaviour or emotional expression prompted a responsible adult to ask, 'what's wrong?' Shelia's defiance of her mother and running away from home could be construed as both a disclosure of her abuse and rebellion to her abuse at home by her Uncle Tom. Second, Shelia tried to disclose her abuse verbally to her mother, but her account was not taken seriously, and so no action was taken by her mother. This led to her morning talk to the class about her abuse by her uncle when her mother disbelieved her, prompting intervention by the teacher, who involved child protection services in undertaking an investigation of CSA.

In terms of her abuse in foster care, she disclosed to her girlfriend, Samantha, who then involved her parents. This disclosure to a trusted peer was also preferred by many young people McElvaney et al. (2014) interviewed. The peer chosen was most often a confident who had 'the experience of mutual sharing of confidences' (McElvaney et al., 2014, p. 116). Shelia was encouraged by her friend, Samantha, to tell her parents what she experienced in foster care, which she did. This brought about the change to safety when Shelia was placed with Samantha and her family as an alternative to another foster care placement.

McElvaney et al. (2014) asked young people who were survivors of CSA what the obstacles and facilitators to disclosure were. These were reported as: being believed, being asked directly about what was wrong and, when they didn't respond, the concerned adult or peer keeping asking.

What stopped disclosure were feeling ashamed of what happened, fears for self and others in the telling and the aftermath of telling, and lack of support of peers for the disclosure (McElvaney et al., 2014, pp. 934–939). Making a difference so that other children would avoid being abused was a strong protective factor in the decision to disclose, according to the young people interviewed (McElvaney et al., 2014).

These findings suggest how complex the process of disclosure of CSA is, between keeping silent, shoring up emotions and internalising the feelings associated with the abuse, and waiting for the relationship or liminal space in which to confide.

The second case study, of Nicky, illustrates the long-term legacy of a survivor who, unlike Shelia, never told anyone about her abuse until she was having parenting issues with her partner in her middle years. She had been seeing her general practitioner because of panic attacks that seemed to be getting worse over recent months, as there was conflict between Debbie and Nicky over the parenting of Nicky's daughter, Taylor. This referral for couple counselling with her partner, Debbie, brought another opportunity to explore Nicky's narrative involving CSA.

Case study: Nicky and Debbie

A general practitioner referred a same-sex couple who were having difficulties with their daughter. The referred client was Nicky, a woman in her mid-40s who had been experiencing escalating panic attacks recently and over the past year. While anti-anxiety medication had been prescribed, as this can have addictive and unwanted side effects, the general practitioner thought other management strategies might be more effective, and so the referral was made to our community mental health centre.

In her background, Nicky came to realise she was a lesbian after having previously been married to an older man she met in her teens. This relationship had been physically abusive, and so Nicky made the decision to leave. After years of living on her own after moving out of this relationship when she reached the age of 25 years, she realised she wanted to have a child. She conceived her daughter, Taylor, with a gay male friend on the understanding that Nicky would take all financial responsibility for raising Taylor but that he would know her as her biological father and take a more detached role in her upbringing.

When Taylor was a toddler, Nicky met and married her girlfriend Debbie, who was ten years older and held a high-ranking position in public services as a manager. Debbie had not had children by choice but felt ready for the role as co-parent, although she realised this would be a new experience for her. Once Debbie joined the family, she took on a co-parenting role with Taylor. It was thought helpful by our clinical director for our family therapy team to see Nicky and Debbie together as a couple to strengthen the couple relationship and encourage them to parent more consistently together. Bowlby (1973), one of the founders of attachment theory, stipulated that, in order to help a child, it was necessary to work with the parents, with the child obtaining parallel support with their own counsellor. Therefore, Taylor was referred to the child and adolescent service to see a counsellor.

Nicky had an earlier history of CSA within her family of origin that had been disclosed to Debbie when their relationship began. A brother who was 13 at the time regularly involved Nicky in acts of oral sex between the ages of seven and nine years when her self-employed parents were looking after their retail business. She did not tell her parents or other adults as she feared it would break up the family and so she coped by turning her emotions inwards and isolating herself, which was noted in her school reports. In particular, her teachers noted that she was absent from school on many occasions and, usually, did not have a note from her parents explaining these periodic absences. She told her teacher she had been sick but there was no one home to care for her and write a sick note because of their business requiring them to work such long hours. No further investigation of the 'sick leave' pattern was made by the teachers.

Given Nicky's early life and background, she was very protective of Taylor, while Debbie had a different style of parenting. During the initial couple session, Nicky described a particular incident that was an example of what the problem was from her perspective. Debbie allowed Taylor to have more freedom as a 16 year old as she had been brought up by more lenient parents who allowed her to attend school discos on weeknights. While Nicky had a curfew for Taylor on weeknights to allow her ample time for sleep and homework and to prepare for school the next day, Debbie thought this was too restrictive for her age and allowed her to go out with school friends until 11 at night to attend a party one weeknight. Taylor did not come home until later than agreed and finally arrived back home with her girlfriends in the early hours of the morning. Her friends said that they had gone home with one of the older men at the party, and he had the idea that they should all 'sleep over' in his bedroom. Taylor and her friends escaped the situation by asking to use the bathroom and fleeing by climbing out of a window. The group of friends felt they had had a 'lucky escape'.

Nicky was very anxious and distressed at Taylor's staying out so late and blamed Debbie for her decision to give Taylor her approval to attend the party on the weeknight without consulting her. It seemed to Nicky that Debbie had not supported her in her parenting. Nicky angrily said to Debbie that 'anything could have happened' to Taylor. In exploring this comment, it was clear that Nicky was reliving some of her own CSA with parents who did not engage with her and so were not seen as confidents. Her parents were often absent from the home because they owned their own retail business and so did not give the children much of their free time. They left their son to 'look after' Nicky. In attachment terms, Nicky had an avoidant style of attachment as her parents were never around after school or at weekends. She looked to her brother as a kind of parental figure because of this.

Debbie apologised for approving Taylor's attendance at the party without consultation and said she would leave the parenting more to Nicky. Next time she agreed that she would support the curfew set by Nicky. This apology allowed Nicky the space to talk about what happened to her with her brother and how alone she felt in not being able to tell anyone what was happening as he was the 'golden haired boy' in the family. Her brother, Dominic, achieved well academically at school and went on to have a successful and comfortable life subsequently. Nicky discussed in the couple sessions the difficulties she had experienced in her family, her subsequent marriage that was physically abusive and life as a single parent. She lacked the education to get a well-paid job and so worked as a preschool assistant so that she would have free child care for Taylor as she worked. She reflected on what she had sacrificed to parent Taylor. The team commended Nicky on the good parenting she had managed despite the many obstacles throughout her life. Taylor, she told Debbie, 'meant everything to her'.

Debbie acknowledged that Nicky had had a rough time in her childhood and in her marriage and described the challenges they faced in the early years of their partnership owing to this. Debbie was encouraging of Nicky to seek help for her educational and career goals by saying she would keep the household finances going to allow her to focus more on her recovery, whatever this involved. Nicky agreed to another couple session in a month's time to review how they were going with the parenting of Taylor.

Implications for practice

Raising teenagers requires a fine balance between encouraging greater independence, a growing sense of their own individuality and the development of relationships with peers and assessing risk and the potential for harm. Survivors of CSA who are parenting can find themselves acting in ways in which they were parented. Alternatively, they might not have a role model for any parenting that they consider healthy. Duncan (1995), in her self-help guide for women disclosing CSA later in life, sees adult survivors on a continuum of parenting styles. At one end of the continuum, the mother may allow the child to do anything at any age, unaware of what is age-appropriate and beneficial to the child's stage of development. This leads to over-expectation and potential risks that the mother may be unaware of. In the example used to illustrate this theme, she describes a client who expected her four year old to care for a two-year-old toddler, as she was unaware of a four year old's needs. She accounts for this as this parent lacking healthy parenting models, which leaves survivors without the knowledge to parent (Duncan, 1995, p. 128). At the other end of the continuum of parenting styles for adult women survivors is when the mother requires total dependence, regardless of the need for individuation and developing relationships outside the home (Duncan, 1995, p. 128). This claustrophobic dependence-inducing style of parenting can be equally harmful. Re-parenting programmes are recommended for adult women survivors as part of their recovery process to enable them to increase their understanding of child development and to begin to trust their own parenting as their knowledge and experience increase (Duncan, 1995, p. 128).

In the example of Nicky and Debbie, they had differing experiences of their own parenting in their respective upbringings. Where one partner is closer to the end of the continuum where freedom and independence are permitted (Debbie), and the other partner is closer to the end of the continuum where protection and restriction are the focus (Nicky), there is the potential for conflict within the relationship over parenting. As Nicky had an avoidant attachment style because there was a lack of boundaries in her family of origin, she was keen to put boundaries and protections in place for her daughter as an expression of her care for Taylor. For the partner who did not have experiences of CSA, as in the case of Debbie, there was a greater tolerance to allow her daughter to exercise her own discretion.

Tables 5.1 and 5.2 summarise the two case studies in terms of risks, protective factors and the major storylines that brought them to therapy as a couple.

Table 5.1 Risk and protective factors in the case of Shelia

Protective factors supporting disclosure as a child	*Risk factors hampering disclosure as a child*	*Life event(s) triggering retelling or re-disclosure*	*Outcome of re-disclosure*
Peer relationships supportive at school Responsible adult believed morning talk and intervened School noticed that something was wrong owing to absences Child protection social workers investigated teacher's concerns	Sexualised contact from uncle continued at home Disbelief by mother when told of uncle's conduct Running away from home	Husband's ill health and fears of him dying and her being left alone. She commented: 'What am I meant to do if you die, I can't find someone else'	Couple counselling strengthened the relationship by exploring the aftermath of CSA Rob witnessed Shelia's healing journey since adolescence
Emotional intelligence – Shelia used her intuition and knew something was 'yukky' about her uncle	Truanting from school Neglect from her mother	Daughters are about to leave home Empty nest syndrome	Shelia parented her daughters allowing for individuation
Finished schooling	Rape in foster care, with threats not to tell anyone	Daughters in teens at similar age when Shelia was abused in foster care	Daughters moved out of home to university
Best friend's family became her own in adolescence	Memory lapses involving CSA continued	Wish for career change	Ties with family of origin, especially mother, severed as an adult
Boyfriend's family support at school and beyond	Dissociation as a coping mechanism	Ongoing contact with in-laws as surrogate family providing an alternative model of family	Royal commission heard her narrative of abuse in foster care

Table 5.2 Risk and protective factors in the case of Nicky

Protective factors supporting disclosure as a child	*Risk factors hampering disclosure as a child*	*Life event(s) triggering retelling or re-disclosure*	*Outcome of re-disclosure*
Learned to detach from family and cope alone Resourceful Isolated as a self-protective strategy	Neglect due to having busy self-employed parents 'Our business comes before the children'	Differences in parenting styles Nicky more protective of her daughter's socialising to limit risk of being abused IPV issues in earlier marriage	Couple counselling strengthened the relationship by exploring the aftermath of CSA

Protective factors supporting disclosure as a child	*Risk factors hampering disclosure as a child*	*Life event(s) triggering retelling or re-disclosure*	*Outcome of re-disclosure*
Attended school but had difficulties concentrating Achieved at school due to intelligence despite absences	Parented by her abuser (brother) Lack of appropriate boundaries in the family	Parallel issues of daughter being of an age where she is wanting more freedom	Identified they had different parenting due to upbringings
Avoidant attachment style	Belief of family that 'what happens in the home remains in the home'	Same-sex couple finding a new model for their parenting	Commitment to partner affirmed
Self sufficient and resourceful	Rigid gender roles at home Easily stressed and ambivalent with peers	Nicky lacked a model for her parenting because of dysfunctional family relationships and disengaged parents	Ties with family of origin, especially mother, severed as an adult
Did not have friends at school	Teachers did not ask directly about absences	Wanted to return to finish her high school education	Greater consultation over parenting

Conclusion

It takes courage for an adult survivor to come forward to inform anyone of their abuse. Disassociation and amnesia can blur the memories of what happened, and, owing to the double betrayal that often features, continuing non-disclosure can be a lifelong theme. This twice-experienced betrayal, by the perpetrator who abuses and the disbelief from the non-abusing caregiver, is another reason for further delays in piecing the fragments of memory into a coherent whole. Retrospective research among survivors has discovered that the disclosure is often paused until middle age. This delay in the disclosure process is more likely when the perpetrator was a close family member rather than a stranger to the child (Wager, 2013). As the case study of Shelia highlights, some early abuse may never be fully remembered owing to the earliness of the CSA and the extent of the abuse, complicated by the tendency towards dissociation and being disbelieved. Raising awareness of the impact of CSA in parenting courses, with appropriate learning materials on how CSA can impact one's parenting, may assist. If the mother or primary caregiver has a history of CSA that is denied, this may make hearing the child difficult, depending what stage the parent/caregiver is at in her own healing from CSA.

A re-telling of the original abuse story and how it impacts thus far is often prompted in the middle years when relationships, health and family undergo many usual life changes. In the case of Shelia, couple counselling was prompted by her partner's health and the anxiety about their future life together. Through couple counselling in which her partner heard her abuse story again, he began to see how their life as a couple had been impacted. He further witnessed how their couple counselling provided the liminal space in which to explore their current patterns of interaction. Second, in the witnessing, they were able to evolve new patterns of interacting that had hitherto been limited by the past CSA narrative. This couple work empowered Shelia to access more of her abuse story and to disclose in a public context. Within the safe crucible of her relationship and home life, she felt able to use this safety as a springboard towards further disclosure in the hope of bringing about personal closure for her and wider social change.

In the next chapter, we move to focusing on the issue of disclosure in the 60+ age group. The focus of this chapter is on the phase of life in which women evolve new understandings of CSA based on putting their experiences in a wider time frame that allows them to look back on earlier years with a transformed personal philosophy and worldview.

References

Bowlby, J. (1973). *Attachment and Loss: Volume 2. Separation: Anxiety and Anger.* Basic Books.

Duncan, K. (1995). *Healing from the Trauma of Childhood Sexual Abuse: The Journey for Women*. Praegar.

Herman, J. (1992). *Trauma and Recovery.* Basic Books.

Jonson, E., & Lindblad, F. (2004). Disclosure, reactions and social support: findings from a sample of adult victims of child sexual abuse. *Child Maltreatment*, 9(2), 190–200.

McElvaney, R. (2015). Disclosure of child sexual abuse: delays, non-disclosure and partial disclosure. What the research tells us and implications for practice. *Child Abuse Review*, 24(3), 159–169. doi:10.1002/car.2280

McElvaney, R., Green, S., & Hogan, D. (2014). To tell or not to tell? Factors influencing young people's informal disclosures of child sexual abuse. *Journal of Interpersonal Violence*, 29(5), 928–947.

Myerhoff, B. G. (1982). *Number our Days: Triumph of Continuity and Culture among Jewish Old People in an Urban Ghetto.* Simon & Schuster/Touchstone Books.

Nasim, R., & Nadan, Y. (2013). Couples therapy with childhood sexual abuse survivors (CSA) and their partners: establishing a context for witnessing. *Family Process*, 52(3), 368–377.

Pack, M. (2002). Sexual abuse counsellors' responses to stress and trauma: a social work perspective. Unpublished PhD thesis. Victoria University of Wellington New Zealand.

Pack, M. (2009). The body as a site of knowing: sexual abuse counsellors' responses to traumatic disclosures. *Women's Studies Journal*, 23(2), 46–56.

Pack, M. (2013). Vicarious traumatisation and resilience: an ecological systems approach to sexual abuse counsellors' trauma and stress. *Sexual Abuse in Australia and New Zealand*, 5(2), 69–76.

Royal Commission of Inquiry. (2024). Royal Commission Hearing into Institutional Responses of State Agencies to Abuse in Care. Retrieved March 2024 from www.abuseincare.org.nz/our-inquiries/royal-commission-hearing-into-institutional-responses-of-state-agencies-to-abuse-in-care/

Thrane. L. E., Yoder, K. A., & Chen, X. (2011). The influence of running away on the risk of female sexual assault in the subsequent year. *Violence and Victims*, 26(6) 818–829.

Turner, V. (1969). Liminality and communitas. In *The Ritual Process: Structure and Anti-Structure* (pp. 41–49). Ithaca, NJ: Cornell University Press.

Wager, N. M. (2013). Sexual revictimization: double betrayal and the risk associated with dissociative amnesia. *Journal of Child Sexual Abuse*, 22(7), 878–899. doi:10.1080/10538712.2013.830666

White, M. (1995). *Re-Authoring Lives: Interviews And Essays.* Adelaide, South Australia: Dulwich Centre.

6 Later years – matured insights integrated into life philosophies, being part of an ageing family and the creation of new memories

> She said 'oh, you must feel really bad … blah blah blah', and I says 'no, actually'. I said 'I'm not a victim anymore. I'm a survivor'. And I said 'I've come back here to make new memories and happy memories'. And that's exactly what I've done.
>
> (Comment made by a research participant interviewed to explore older women's reflections on their CSA later in their lives; Graham et al., 2022, p. 712)

Introduction

In this chapter, the issues for women survivors who are in the 60+ age range are explored. With increasing longevity, there are more women in this age group coming forward to deal with their recollections of sexual abuse. By the age of 60+, they may be less constrained by the taboos from earlier decades in which CSA was less openly discussed. If their CSA has been dismissed as an inappropriate subject to discuss, this can be a time when it may be more possible to address it. As in the comment above, made by an adult woman reflecting on her life narrative, there is often a desire to look beyond victimhood to see oneself living outside a compromised life, to be seen more as an active participant in shaping one's current life, which includes looking forward to the future. There is an appreciation that, though one's early life may have been marred by the many effects of the abuse and the need to keep it secret within the family, with the passage of time there is a 're-authoring' of one's earlier life (White, 1995). In the comment above, the research participant was strongly challenging the perceptions of others. This belief that a history of childhood sexual abuse tarnishes the whole of life irrevocably is challenged by more optimistic revisions of the past. The research participant quoted by Graham et al. (2022) wanted others to know that she had transformed early adversity into a safe, happy and enjoyable phase of life by a shift of home location to where she grew up. Although this location was once closely linked to her abuse, she felt she could return there to live, spelling a break from the old life to the new.

DOI: 10.4324/9781032669205-6

Themes prevalent in the 60+ era of life intersect with the culmination of this healing process. Usual themes for women in this age range typically include the care of grandchildren and elderly parents, concerns about descendants across the generations, health and financial challenges. A growing sense of spirituality and planning for the end of life may also feature. These broader life themes are juxtaposed with the healing journey of women survivors of CSA. Disclosure of earlier histories of abuse can be seen as a means of tackling 'unfinished business' during this phase of life, where there is a looking back over the entirety of one's life with developed insights and the application of personal philosophies as a lens through which one can begin to overview one's life as a whole. The spiritual and cultural aspects of believing in an afterlife after death in some shape or form are other issues to be addressed when working with women survivors in this era of their lives. For example, in my clinical practice, I have commonly encountered survivors who express fears of being reunited with perpetrators who have passed after the survivor's death. These fears and the woman's own spiritual beliefs need space to be discussed and to be creatively explored. Such a case from my own clinical practice will be discussed to conclude this chapter.

Themes from the research literature on 60+ women survivors of CSA

There are a number of identifiable themes for women CSA survivors in the 60+ age range in terms of circumstances that may reawaken their CSA issues and their legacy. These themes include: difficulties self-advocating when navigating health and social service systems for the health care that survivors of CSA need; membership in an ageing family, responsibility for the care of elderly parents and, ultimately, the death of family members, including the perpetrator(s) of CSA and the non-offending parent; the growth of spirituality; and a search for a community in which to gain a sense of belonging. These themes will be illustrated with a case study drawing from my clinical practice.

Navigating health care systems and finding appropriate care

The research literature suggests that, during later stages of life, often referred to as 'the senior years', health issues can emerge that interface with the need for specialised medical and rehabilitation services. Some of these health concerns are seen as being linked to the aftermath of CSA. For example, Lee et al. (2014) discovered that childhood trauma can lead to metabolic syndrome (MetS) in abuse survivors as they age, leading to negative health trajectories and outcomes if undiagnosed and untreated (Lee et al., 2014). The authors found that the risk of developing MetS was higher for women survivors of CSA than for men. They identified specific psychosocial pathways to account for the association. Women who had a history of CSA were more likely to have poor sleep quality, leading to sleep disorders, and stress-related eating, leading to higher BMI. MetS symptoms were more prevalent for women survivors of

CSA owing to these stress-related behaviours that were a consequence of an unhealthy lifestyle with long-term impacts on health (Lee et al., 2014).

Dealing with the disclosure of CSA concurrently with a major health issue can complicate the seeking of health care and impact the physical healing and treatment trajectory. For example, there may be concerns about receiving health services when residential care is needed. As women live on average several years longer than men, globally, they are more prone to the diseases of old age such as dementia. Elders who have developed dementia were found to be more at risk of abuse, in various kinds of care situations, compared to those without a diagnosis of dementia. The perpetrator of their subsequent abuse was more often a person known to them (family member, caregiver or another nursing home resident) than a stranger (Burgess & Phillips, 2006). Those elders who were abused presented behaviour cues of distress rather than verbal disclosures. They were easily confused and verbally manipulated and were more often victim to being physically abused and beaten. Perpetrators who were identified by abused elders with dementia had less chance of being brought to the notice of authorities because of the elders' capacities (Burgess & Phillips, 2006).

Rajan and colleagues (2021) investigated the relationship between patients with a history of abuse and their health care-seeking behaviours in the Swedish context. They found that the majority of patients were women with CSA histories. Eighty-two per cent of the patients surveyed had experienced problems accessing health care appropriate to their needs. The authors concluded that there is both a gender equity issue and a social justice concern that victims of historical sexual abuse do not receive the health care they need in later years. The authors concluded that women CSA survivors are prone to getting lost when navigating complex specialist health care systems (Rajan et al., 2021). As long-term health issues have been associated with childhood sexual abuse, the legacy of which often clarifies in later life, delays in obtaining appropriate health care in a timely manner can have far-reaching consequences in the 60+ age group. These findings suggest vulnerabilities of adult survivors who are elders to being misunderstood, leading to a sense of being missed or even re-abused in later life. Not being understood or believed when having their health issues investigated or treated in a timely way can mirror being disbelieved as a child or adolescent when they attempted to disclose abuse. The main obstacle to disclosure of CSA to health care professionals has been found to be the issue of time, with consultants under pressure indicating it would take much longer to explore CSA as part of the consultation (McGregor et al., 2010). Being comfortable with hearing disclosure of CSA and having adequate training in trauma-informed theory are other considerations for the professional development of health care professionals (McGregor et al., 2010).

The search for inner strength and resolution

The research literature reviewed in earlier chapters had found that it takes a survivor a varying number of years before she discloses that she has been abused. The consensus is that it is often not until the middle years of life that the right constellation of confiding relationships presents to foster disclosure (McElvaney, 2015; Mooney & McGregor, 2018). Earlier chapters have explored some of the facilitators and some of the barriers to disclosure, which include fear of further abuse, fear of splitting the family up, cultural taboos and reprisals from significant others if they disclose (Alaggia et al., 2019; Brazelton, 2011; Brazelton, 2015). The finding that childhood sexual abuse happens in a context and can involve a complex interplay of individual intrapsychic factors, such as anxiety, depression, dissociation, PTSD and interpersonal factors, means it is unsurprising that women delay talking to anyone about their CSA. The relational barriers to disclosure include threats of re-victimisation by the perpetrator and the presence of interlocking forms of abuse such as physical, emotional and psychological (Halvorsen et al., 2020).

The findings from interviewing older women about their processes of healing from a history of CSA identified that women in later years seek some form of resolution, either by reframing earlier interpretations of what happened, by developing a sense of agency over disclosure or by deciding whom to tell and how much to tell.

An understanding of what is needed for each woman to recover and transform her experiences to allow for an integration of CSA trauma into her life's narrative was the topic of investigation for a group of researchers in the New Zealand context. Graham et al. (2022) undertook a longitudinal study of women survivors of CSA in the 60+ age range. Their interviews with women highlighted that some women, over the 25 years of the longitudinal study, did not disclose their CSA to anyone except the researchers, yet they had a philosophical view of their CSA, and most had moved on from their grieving (Graham et al., 2022). Developing agency over to whom, when and where older women survivors of CSA choose to disclose was also discovered by the same group of researchers. Their participants were aged from 60 to 80 years of age, with an average age of 71 (Graham et al., 2022). The women interviewed were asked about the effects CSA had had on their lives and the role that CSA had in their life in the present. The strategies that had helped them to heal and move on with their lives were investigated during in-depth interviews over the duration of the study. Not all the women had disclosed CSA to any person other than to the researcher, but this disclosure and the follow-up interview were significant to the women as they were found to help their healing from CSA (Graham et al., 2022). The authors found that most of the women survivors interviewed over the 25-year period were able to make sense of their abuse by reinterpreting what had happened and attaching new meaning to their CSA and their relationship with the perpetrator of their abuse. They were able to evolve strategies that enabled them to think about their abuse less frequently and to feel more in charge of the decision to disclose. They were more able to decide on the process of how to disclose, when to disclose and to whom to disclose (Graham et al., 2022). Three themes were present in the healing processes of the women interviewed. The first was how their self-perception had been impacted by the CSA. The second was how their perceptions of others and of their relationships had been impacted (being cautious in relationships with men) and whom they trusted. Third, most participants felt their experiences of CSA had negatively impacted their self-esteem, which led to doubts about themselves and their sense of self-worth in the world up to this point in their life (Graham et al., 2022). However, they found the opportunity to be interviewed about their experiences of CSA over the years of the study had developed their relationships with the researchers, which were now very important to them.

The act of speaking about CSA, aloud or in writing, has been compared to an act of destroying one's past, including memories of childhood (Halvorsen et al., 2020). However, as the opening quotation in this chapter, from an older woman with a CSA background, indicates, it can also be an act of re-creation and of building a new life narrative based on new memories that are happier than those that have been experienced in the past. As we have seen in previous chapters, how the original disclosure was met by others is influential in decisions about whether and how to disclose again to others. The balance of protective factors existing with risk factors continues to impact the recovery process and healing trajectory in later years.

The relationship with the abuser and nature and severity/duration of the abuse can be buffered by a secure attachment to a non-offending caregiver or significant other, and this can assist in the recovery process. Engaging in new meaning-making activities to re-author a new life narrative and making new memories was a means of freeing oneself from early childhood experiences are prominent in this phase of the life cycle.

Finding confiding relationship(s)

If a safe attachment has not been possible throughout adulthood, women survivors can find it difficult to trust health professionals, and this can influence the healing journey for those who develop illness, which is more commonly encountered in this phase of life. For example, women with a history of CSA who are sufferers of long-term health conditions were found to have less favourable treatment journeys through the health services owing to difficulties engaging with their doctors, nurses and other health professionals (McGregor et al., 2010). The relationships with multiple health professionals needed to navigate health systems that are often uncoordinated and confusing often triggered the challenges of forming trust in a relationship and being let down by the health care provider. This kind of experience has the potential for rekindling the experience of being mistreated or abused (McGregor et al., 2010). Flashpoints of challenge for women survivors of CSA undergoing treatment included boundary violations involved in the contact with the woman's body during such procedures as scanning and diagnostic work-up, surgeries, chemotherapy and radiotherapies, for example.

For elder women survivors of CSA whose therapists are also women survivors of CSA, the latter advocate the writing of a life memoir that contextualises the conflicting emotions women experience now as elders. In her account of assisting a woman client she refers to as 'Ruth', psychotherapist Jean Walbridge reconnects with her own experiences of abuse 60 years prior to understand where the resistances are in their therapeutic work together (Walbridge, 2021). Speaking aloud to a therapist or writing down what happened and the feelings related to one's recollections of CSA can be a revealing therapeutic process that can ultimately be transformative.

One of the most difficult issues to disclose to another is the admission that the sexual contact made them feel special or there were aspects that were enjoyed as they became normalised over time. This theme of disclosing what happened in an attempt to heal the inner child during the later years of life can again become a priority, as Walbridge explains:

> I am finally able to experience Ruth's grief with her – the grief at the loss of a tabooed connection with a loved brother – and I am able to normalize that experience, speaking softly with to her, defining her reaction as a conditioned response. Perhaps the cruellest aspect of adult–child sexual abuse is the murder of innocence, the forced arousal of feelings in a child for which they are not prepared and which ought to be their privilege to develop in their own time and with other people of their own choosing.
>
> (Walbridge, 2021, p. 128)

As both Walbridge and her client had experiences of pleasure during arousal as part of their abuse, they both were dealing with confusion and guilt about their abuse. Grieving for their innocence was the focus for both Walbridge and Ruth during this phase of their recovery from CSA.

The socio-cultural background of the individual woman in elder years is also important to acknowledge as colouring the context. Findings from Brazelton's (2011) narrative research using a storyboarding approach with older women in the 40–70 age group indicate that there are several factors that influence the act of disclosure and, therefore, the healing trajectory post-disclosure for older women.

First, Brazelton speaks to the historical and cultural stereotypes relating to African American women. She sees such cultural and familial stereotypes as stemming from slavery and the perceptions of African American family. These stereotypes, which are prominent owing to North America's history of white colonialism, influence the disclosure of historical CSA for elderly women survivors who are of African American background (Brazelton, 2011; Brazelton, 2015). Second, Brazelton discovered that a lack of language and comprehension due to the early stage of development during which the abuse occurred can also affect meaning making and disclosure. Third, the findings of Brazelton's study suggest that the act of disclosing or telling another about her CSA does not necessarily result in the woman's healing. However, the act of disclosure to another is considered to be part of the trajectory towards healing. Brazelton, therefore, has a chronological, biographical view of disclosure as a lifelong process. The study concludes that, for African American women, telling another what happened in relation to CSA extends long past the initial experience of disclosure (Brazelton, 2011; Brazelton, 2015). Accounts of what happened in terms of CSA recollections can also change over the life course, which can be apparent by the elder years of life (Brazelton, 2011; Brazelton, 2015). To concur with this research, remembering one's CSA, as we have seen, can be a gradual process depending on the facilitators of and barriers to disclosure mentioned throughout this book.

Lastly, Brazelton's research discusses the notion of 'reconciliation' with the sexual abuse across the life course. This reconciliation is seen as helpful for women CSA survivors to be able to engage in positive caregiving experiences with parents and family members as it frees women to attend to matters in the present rather than these being continually overlaid with the past (Brazelton, 2011; Brazelton, 2015). Dealing with family members who are ageing and in need of care can bring survivors into closer proximity with their perpetrators, and this is the subject of the next theme in the literature.

Dealing with an ageing family and caring for parents who are terminally ill or dying

The need to revisit an earlier history of CSA can also be triggered by the caring for a parent in older age and, ultimately, facing the death of a parent or other primary caregiver. This can be emotionally triggering if the parent is a perpetrator of the CSA, or if women survivors are brought into contact with family when family members have previously disbelieved disclosures of abuse. In this caregiving role with a terminally ill parent, there can be a mourning for the loss of the family one had expected to have in this stage of life or the letting go of this expectation. For example, in her interviews with women in this age group who had histories of CSA with their older brothers and were dealing with the caring for or anticipating the loss of their parent(s), Monahan reminds us of the importance of dealing with the feelings related to historical CSA during such times (Monahan, 2010). Issues for the women interviewed by Monahan included being brought into contact with an older brother who had abused them in their childhood through the needs of their ill or dying parent (Monahan, 2010). The ages at which her research participants had experienced their abuse ranged from nine to early teens. The brothers who sexually abused the women interviewed were at least five years older. Three were stepbrothers, with other perpetrators being biological brothers. The abuse experienced was on the 'severe spectrum', ranging from genital fondling to intercourse and oral sex. This abuse occurred on a frequent and regular basis of at least two to three times per month (Monahan, 2010, p. 363). All of the women participants who were interviewed had been in therapy for sibling sexual abuse previously. The women discussed how the historical CSA affected their current relationships with their siblings and their functioning in daily life. The lasting legacy of CSA was realised in this phase of life. The ways in which the dynamics of their family relationships had been permanently damaged by the CSA were discussed, and these dynamics continued in the present. Being brought into contact with the abuser over the care of a parent raised old ways of relating between brother and sister. The brother's bullying and threatening behaviour towards his sister was noted in their adult dealings with one another. The issue of a parent disbelieving the woman and favouring the son, which had kept the CSA going in the family, continued in the adult interactions, as the following comment illustrates:

> Even when my father was dying and we had hospice at the house, my mother still protected my brother. I knew I could never tell her (about the abuse) because I was afraid she would have a heart attack or collapse on the floor, plus all the stress with my father. Yet I was running around doing everything and he was still doing his drugs. I wanted to scream and tell her what happened – 'he's not your "angel"' – but what good would that do?
> (Monahan, 2010, p. 364)

Wanting their non-abusing parent or guardian to acknowledge their abuse was a belief deeply held by all of the participants in this study, regardless if they felt they could, and even had, told them of their CSA. The CSA issues became prominent again at the bedside of the dying parent, but, owing to the dynamics of the family, four of the nine women interviewed had never disclosed their abuse to anyone in their family of origin. Saying what had happened in another context was important to the women interviewed, and to realistically appraise what they could achieve in changing their family of origin's functioning. This realisation was important going forward from this experience (Monahan, 2010, p. 365).

When a family system cannot be expected to believe the women survivor, even in her 60s and beyond, there can be a searching for an inner place of peace within herself in which the issues related to CSA can be processed intrapsychically. Alternative support systems, such as therapy groups, and spiritual development are often features for women survivors in later years, as we will now move on to explore.

Searching for belonging in a community

The transformational potential is enhanced for many women in the 60+ age range by being freed from the shackles of full-time employment or moving into part-time employment, retiring or giving up work, or moving to a rural location to find a better balance between work and other pursuits. These were themes of my earlier research with sexual abuse counsellors, many of whom were in this age range and the majority of whom were survivors of CSA (Pack, 2010). Over many years of doing their own personal therapy on their CSA, they had found ways of balancing the rigours of work with their own healing as they worked with women survivors who were dealing with their CSA. In interviews with 30 experienced sexual abuse therapists, I discovered as a theme the search for inner strength through spirituality. This was not associated with organised religion, as one of my participants who had been a minister of religion said. She had left the church hierarchy because of its patriarchal structures and being exposed to stories of abuse within her church. She had decided it was not ethical to remain in that role as CSA within the church came to light, and she was asked to serve on a disciplinary board.

In another of my interviews with sexual abuse counsellors who were also survivors of CSA, another counsellor participant had joined a spiritual community to move beyond organised religion to a daily spiritual practice with like-minded others. She explains the value of community in the following excerpt from my interview with her:

> I value currently and for the past twenty years, being part of a community of people with similar spiritual beliefs … their work is to carry out spiritual retreat work. And as my own spirituality has grown and changed, I still feel comfortable with that group of women. Probably half are Catholic but half are not. I feel valued and accepted for the person I am having moved away from Catholicism.
>
> (Pack, 2002, p. 229)

This comment mirrors another older woman's account of her searching for inner sanctuary by periodically going on retreat at a monastery to live as one of the monks, spending days in silent meditation and prayer. Through such inner reflection in a supportive community of spiritual beings, Leibrich describes finding a place within her that she recognised had existed throughout her life, and so was familiar, but which she did not yet know. In the years of patient spiritual reflection, she found that what she was looking for was there throughout her life, awaiting her discovery in the years before her death in her early 70s (Leibrich, 2015). Disclosure of CSA may settle in this liminal space, through such practices and with such a supportive framework, to allow life to go on, albeit in new ways.

But living in a community is not always a positive experience for all women, as it was for the survivors above. Those children who grew up in communes of the 1960s and 1970s, who are now aged in their 50s and 60s, were often exposed to adverse circumstances such as the widely reported sexual abuse (Gibson et al., 2011). Gibson et al. (2011), in their follow-up study of adult survivors of CSA at the Centrepoint commune, explored the experiences of child residents, now adults, who had grown up in that context. Their research participants reported psychological harm that came from a variety of sources, including parental neglect, drug use and involvement in sexual activity from the age of three years. This study highlights the ways in which a cluster of risk factors can leave children and young people vulnerable to the misuse of adult power and involvement in adult sexuality. The risk of CSA is heightened when there are a lack of appropriate boundaries, and safe adult relationship. In the case of Centrepoint whose child victims have since applied for therapy and redress for their loss of childhood, it has left those survivors with a lack of modelling of safe relationships and attachment to a consistent caregiver (Gibson et al., 2011).

The grief of CSA held for so long by senior years can create a need for expression again in another attempt at finding the way forward in a life forever changed by earlier experiences. The main obstacles to disclosure in the 60+ age range have been found to be the age when the abuse occurred (the earliness of the abuse) and the era in which it occurred, which for older women was characterised by sexual abuse being a taboo issue not to be discussed. Reflecting upon my clinical practice in the 60+ age range of women survivors of CSA brings to mind my practice with a 71-year-old woman who was dealing with a terminal cancer diagnosis and the life and death issues such a diagnosis brings up. As she was navigating the complex treatment for her condition, she was concurrently looking back at her life and her lifelong journey of healing from CSA.

Case study: Alice's story

Alice sought compensation for her experiences of CSA by telephoning a government-funded national helpline I had worked on that gave survivors of CSA information about the process of lodging a claim for mental injury for past sexual abuse incident(s). The helpline also took responsibility for informing survivors of their entitlement once the claim was accepted. At first contact, Alice thought she might like to lodge a sensitive claim, but, as we talked, she realised she wished to tell her ex-partner and family what had happened to her in her childhood as an expression of her grief at her lost childhood and early adulthood. Looking back at her life, she could now see that much of her adult life had been lived in a limited way as a consequence of her CSA.

Alice, aged 71 years, told me that she had come to an age where she felt she had learned much about what was important to her in her life. On her 70th birthday, she made the decision to disclose what had happened to her as a child and also made her the person she was today. She had a plan for disclosure to her family as a means of establishing a resolution by putting the past in perspective. The need for disclosure was prompted when she was told she had a terminal cancer diagnosis and had, at best, a couple of years to live, despite having chemotherapy in her late 60s. Although she was offered further treatment, she found the intrusion of having to attend hospitals and clinics for days upon end wasteful of her limited time left and so she had decided to stop all treatment. As a deeply spiritual woman, she felt she wanted to make a stand as an adult so that her close family members knew what she had endured during her childhood. She had thought about writing her adult children a letter of disclosure to be read after her demise, but then considered this would not address dealing with the aftermath from her family who would have their own issues about their relative, who was uncle to her children. She had decided to host a meeting with her ex-husband and her adult sons on her parents' farm, where one of her children still lived, to let them know what had happened to her with her brother many years ago. She mainly wanted to tell them about how the experience of CSA impacted her life on and off when the original recollections were triggered by key life events and milestones. She said that she hadn't always remembered what happened, but memories gradually emerged over time. Deciding to tell her abuse story was a brave decision, but she had developed a sense of agency over the process of disclosure now that issues of sexual abuse were more openly discussed and not taboo, as her parents' and her own generation believed they should be. She saw this as her final opportunity to tell selected family members about her experience. She also added that she wished to apologise to them if she had sometimes seemed far away when they needed her to be present and responsive earlier in their lives.

Alice thought about what she wanted to disclose. She didn't want to go into the detail of what had happened, but rather to tell her sons, who were themselves parents, more about the context of how it all happened and what the ongoing impact had been during her life. She was hoping to start a conversation about what they had noticed about her when they were growing up and to get some idea of what they might have surmised about her ongoing relationship with their uncle. Her sons, now in their 40s and 50s, had families and partners of their own, and so she thought she could have an adult conversation with them now, a conversation she thought she could never have had earlier in their lives.

She recollected that early abuse by her brother when she was aged six to eight years became more of an issue during adolescence. She thought their 'games together' were part of usual child play until then. When she began socialising with teen peers whose boyfriends and first kisses were discussed by them as milestones to be cherished rather than dreaded, she thought about her CSA again. She recalls asking her girlfriends if they had been kissed when they were younger, but her friends didn't understand what she was trying to say. As they did not have an experience of CSA, they had no framework for understanding what she had endured during her childhood.

Alice's adult years: late teens to 30s

Alice had met her husband at 17 years and married and quickly had children, so that she had three sons under the age of five by the time she was in her mid-20s. She had never told anyone about what had happened with her brother and had 'swept the memories under the carpet'. At the time, she didn't think disclosure to anyone was an option. It was not until she was herself a parent that she felt the early recollections of abuse emerge again and realised that she had married early as a way of getting as far as she could away from her family of origin. She further realised, in her full-time homemaker role, that she didn't find that life as a stay-at-home mother to be very fulfilling and longed to return to complete some form of tertiary education.

When she had separated from her husband, she found satisfaction in her new lifestyle of working part time while co-parenting her sons with him. She had found ways to cope with her CSA by reframing her experiences with her brother as his involving her in games being 'special'. She more recently had seen his behaviour as an attempt to take advantage of her vulnerability as his younger sibling who did not know anything about adult sexuality. When she was a child, what he did was seen by her as being mostly 'yukky' and 'weird' at the time. There were parts of her childhood, she said, she had blocked out and could not remember. She couldn't recall telling anyone about the abuse as a child, but she was not sure if she tried telling her mother or not. What she mainly recalls is the feeling of dread about the 'games' played by her brother. I noticed there were long periods of silence when she was telling me about what had happened. I also noticed how she negated the legacy of her abuse and even what had happened.

Sorsoli (2010, p. 136) talks about the disclosures of women survivors of CSA in this age group as often as involving 'smokescreens' and 'evasions'. Women survivors who were interviewed for her research clearly stated they had been abused, but they were sometimes uncertain about having told anyone about their CSA. This tendency to avoid this discussion seemed to be an avoidance of the whole issue of who knew about the CSA. The question of who the significant others were to whom they had disclosed was the most difficult issue for the women research participants to discuss with the researchers. There seemed confusion among the women interviewed about how their mothers could not have known what happened (Sorsoli, 2010, p. 136). Therefore, there was an implicit belief that their mothers would have known without their being told. The implication of this research finding is that women survivors may believe they have disclosed even though they have not. This is because of the belief that mothers intuitively know what is happening with their children, and, therefore, the survivor should not have had to tell her in this worldview. Another possible explanation for this assumption is that it avoids the issue of disclosure by the women, so avoiding the feeling of vulnerability associated with attracting a negative response from the person disclosed to (Sorsoli, 2010).

The ending of the call from Alice

I invited Alice to phone me if she had decided what she wanted to do with her healing, as counselling for her past CSA would be available if she wished. She thanked me for this but felt counselling or psychotherapy was not what she needed at this point in her life as she had 'coped by doing' things to change her life. She asked if she could telephone me once she had talked things over with her adult sons and her ex-partner, who was still a part of the family, to let me know how this meeting went. Alice was nervously anticipating the conversation to be a very difficult one. I indicated that she would be welcome to re-contact me through the freephone helpline and I wished her well with the meeting. The initial contact made me consider what survivors of CSA needed in the 60+ age range, and the fact that counselling and psychotherapy were not the priority for some older women who had come to terms with their abuse through attributing blame to the perpetrator and parental neglect. Alice had spent much of her earlier life blaming herself for allowing the abuse to happen because it made her feel special and attached in the relationship with her brother when parental neglect coloured her home life and relationship with her parents.

Reflections on the case of Alice

Although I never met Alice in person and only talked with her by telephone, I had nevertheless managed to build a connection. It was a promising sign, I thought, that Alice felt encouraged to contact me again. I had provided a safe container as a virtual stranger who was offering her support to do whatever she felt she needed to do to recover from her past experiences of CSA. Reflecting on that contact with Alice more recently, it made me think of the teleconsultations prevalent during the COVID-19 pandemic, and I concluded that there is much that can be done by telephone and using online technologies. Even though my contact with Alice was in pre-COVID-19 years, there were advantages to having a national freephone number that had a helping professional at the end of it. The anonymity of talking with an available, empathetic professional by telephone might be less challenging for some women than a formal appointment with face-to-face contact in an office setting. This is particularly so for those women survivors who experienced disbelief and social stigma surrounding their abuse owing to their families reaction and the taboos and morals of the time in which they were abused, and were worried that someone might see them coming to see a counsellor if they lived in a small town or rural area.

For Alice, and the majority of the women interviewed by Graham et al. (2022), the recollections of CSA as an older woman did not bring forth the same emotional expression that they did in earlier years, when sadness and grief for a lost childhood predominated and were felt more intensely. Anger was noted for those participants where there was a felt absence of justice being achieved for the survivor by the perpetrator being brought to the authorities to account for their actions. Being let down by one or both parents featured in this anger and hurt at their lack of intervention to stop the abuse. For a few of the women interviewed, these issues left them with a sense of unfinished business related to their CSA that endured (Graham et al., 2022).

The follow-up phone call

Alice did call me back some weeks later to tell me what she had decided to do with counselling for her abuse and in relation to lodging a sensitive claim. I suggested that she write down her experiences of CSA as a way of hearing herself express what happened in words, as this can sometimes be helpful in deciding what to do next. When she called me back, she had written this memoir I recount to you now. She had decided to read it to her sons and ex-husband at a gathering she had organised. One of her sons reacted by weeping at hearing what their mother had endured as a child. She was also able to express that, at times, she had not wanted the games played with her brother. Instead, she wanted them to stop, as they felt sometimes like a poor substitute for the attention and care that should, in retrospect, have come from her parents rather than a sibling. Now, as an elder reflecting on her life, she feels her brother also needed closer parenting and so was deprived, as she was, of appropriate parenting in that sense. Alice told her gathered family that she wanted to explain, rather than apologise for, the way that the CSA had made her distant and stressed, as it had affected her life intermittently ever since. She was able to express why she launched into marriage early to escape her family of origin. She was no longer afraid of any possible negative consequences of telling them this as her time frame for life was now limited by cancer. Since her diagnosis, every moment seemed precious and an opportunity not to be missed.

Her sons were very upset at the news but it also brought them resolution. They did feel their mother's unhappiness during their upbringing, which they had construed as their mother being unhappy in her marriage to their father. Her ex-partner said he had surmised she had some experience of abuse in her family having met her family of origin and noticed the interaction between them being strained when they first married. He said he was aware of why she wanted to move geographically as far away as possible, yet he was confused as to why this did not mean a break from her past and the beginning of a new life. He now understood the failure of the relationship better and said that he was sad that he had not known all of this earlier. He had since gone on to have another relationship and further children. He had always co-parented but never understood what Alice's concerns were about their relationship and blamed himself for not doing enough to salvage the relationship. He thanked Alice for taking the time to tell him what had happened.

Table 6.1 gives a summary of the risks and protective factors that operated in Alice's life, preventing disclosure in the past, and the current protective factors that facilitated a first telling in the present.

Table 6.1 Risk and protective factors in the case of Alice

Protective factors supporting disclosure as a child	*Risk factors hampering disclosure as a child*	*Life event(s) triggering a retelling or re-disclosure*	*Outcome of re-disclosure*
Came to see the behaviour of her brother as being 'sexual abuse' Anxious-ambivalent attachment style as rejected by mother although she had tried to tell her about CSA	Shame No one talked about those topics Anticipated not being believed Brother favoured by mother Mother disbelieved her disclosure of CSA saying 'Children need to experiment'	Cancer diagnosis Terminal illness Uncertainty about the future Reviewing her earlier life	Formal disclosure to her family – sons and ex-partner Support from her sons and ex-husband

Protective factors supporting disclosure as a child	*Risk factors hampering disclosure as a child*	*Life event(s) triggering a retelling or re-disclosure*	*Outcome of re-disclosure*
Realised her family patterns of communication and interaction were dysfunctional	Social taboos existing that prevented talking about abuse openly in the 1950s when Alice was a child Left school early without finishing high school	Birth of first grandchild	Unfinished business addressed to some extent
Realised her mother would not listen to her	CSA normalised as being usual	Returned to education when separated from her marriage	Positive response from family
Belief and hope that others outside the family might believe her one day	Family of origin was tightly knit and insular, had few contacts with neighbours or local community	Left home early to marry Parents and abuser dead	Hoping to avoid intergenerational legacy of CSA in the welcoming of a new grandchild
Knew she would be better off once she was able to leave home	Anticipated that her mother would favour her brother	Feeling of 'moving on' past her abuse	

Discussion

This case study mirrors the findings of an earlier research describing how women survivors have different ways of remembering. In a qualitative study of women survivors of CSA, one theme was that they recovered memories of CSA gradually, having 'forgotten' these memories for many years. The second theme was that others interviewed continued to have partial recall or incomplete memories of CSA (Sorsoli, 2010, p. 133). All interviewed wanted to remain silent about these recollections as a kind of self-preservation, as well as to avoid disruptions in key relationships. The process of remembering seemed to occur spontaneously for the women interviewed, all participants finding it somewhat hard to explain how specifically they had recalled but commenting that they had not always had the recollections of CSA that they had when interviewed. Usually, there were life events that prompted the arising of recollections of CSA. Motherhood was one of these events, and another involved intimate relationship issues. In the safety of a counselling relationship, one woman discussed a piecing together of hitherto incoherent flashbacks that formed a narrative which seemed to come together 'out of the blue' (Sorsoli, 2010, p. 133).

Dissociation, as illustrated in earlier chapters, may be dependent on the nature of the response to the abuse from others. The shame and betrayal that are a legacy of not being believed have been conceptualised as a 'double betrayal' (Wager, 2013). The relationship to the perpetrator, including a close parental one, is reported as being a common reason for silence. The internalisation of the abuse being their fault was found to be prevalent in the women's earlier decades of life (Wager, 2013, p. 883).

As Sorsoli's research (2010) was conducted with four women in their 20s and 30s, its findings contrast with the longitudinal research of Graham et al.'s (2022) study of women in the 60–80 age group. Graham et al. (2022) found that women in the 60+ age range remembered much detail about what happened in their childhood and details of whom they told or did not tell about their CSA during earlier decades. This may be accounted for by long-term memory becoming more prominent later in life. Most participants had moved out of anger and rage about their CSA into a philosophical perspective about what had happened to them in childhood. They saw the perpetrator as being limited in their understanding of the consequences of their actions, and so the women survivors of CSA, to some extent, developed a degree of compassion for them. A survivor narrative had evolved by these later decades of life that was serving to put the past in the past so that their life in the present seemed richer and less limited by CSA than they recalled it having been in earlier decades (Graham et al., 2022).

The case study of Alice reflects these findings in that she had denied her CSA until a relationship break brought her life narrative into sharper focus. She was then able to see how her life had been impacted by the CSA experience. She realised that the legacy of being abused by her brother and not being able to discuss this with anyone had meant that parts of her life were avoided or forgotten as a way of dealing with the aftermath of the abuse. In her 70s, in the midst of dealing with a major health crisis, a terminal diagnosis, she began to think about the importance of her adult relationships to her and in her healing journey from CSA. She did not want therapy but had decided that she wanted to explain some things about her early life to these family members. She felt gratitude for the significant others in her adult life and realised her emotional engagement with them was limited in earlier decades owing to the hidden parts of her experience and the ongoing pain of CSA. She found disclosure to her family at her stage of life to be both an explanation and a 'putting right', as their wife and parent.

Conclusion

The findings from earlier chapters that discuss how CSA has impacted women's lives at key milestones are beneficial to an ongoing processing of memories and emotional responses through the disclosure of CSA and its effects over time. Aligning with earlier chapters, healing from CSA is a gradual awakening process that can be derailed when the survivor is not listened to or when there are other obstacles to disclosure that are having an impact, such as societal or cultural taboos about CSA. In the 60+ age range, this can be a time of seeing one's life on a broader canvas. As the case study of Alice illustrates, elder years often bring to fruition a reframing of the event that enables wider disclosure, which involves risk taking to trust others with a CSA story. In particular, Alice was able to see her brother's abuse in the context of parental neglect and grief about the mothering or parenting that was not available for the formation of a secure attachment when she and her brother were children. While not accepting of the CSA, Alice's priority was to develop an alternative account of what had happened subsequently in her life, with her goal to marry early to separate from parents who did not protect her from the abuse. Her family of origin did not provide the safe relationship in which she could have ever disclosed as she saw it. Her parents were now both deceased and so were not present to have this conversation retrospectively. Disclosure and the timing of it come to be seen more as an opportunity not to be missed when family members, including the perpetrator of the abuse, are nearing the end of life. Alternatively, if deceased, as they were in Alice's family, the CSA narrative may be told to others.

The historical times the survivor has lived through may have had overarching social taboos that prevented the disclosure of abuse, which was the reason for Alice deciding to make time to discuss the aftermath of what had happened with her sons and ex-partner. She didn't want therapy or counselling, as she had come to terms with what had happened through changing the course of her life after she left her marriage, which she felt had limited her personal growth. She then decided to return to the education that she felt deprived of because of her CSA and the need to escape her family of origin.

Helping professionals could apply this reframing process when working with this age group to ask survivors how they navigated key choice points in their lives, such as relationships, obtaining education, career and having their own children. Retrospectively, women have learned much from earlier experiences and, in the 60+ era, are living at a time when the stigma of CSA would have hopefully reduced. By the time women seek help for their issues of childhood sexual abuse, they have navigated many hurdles to achieve what they wish to do in life. They have amassed knowledge over decades, and this reservoir of knowledge can be reflected on and applied to inform current decision making and action as well as to plan for the future. The cultural background of women survivors and how the healing journey from CSA differs within and across cultures are gaps in the existing literature and are areas for future research.

Alice did telephone me back to tell me how things had gone with her family gathering. From her perspective, it had brought a sense of relief that things not said had now been said. Her aim was to have this conversation and then leave it open for her family to connect with her on the issues, which they did, and this brought forth more support from them. By talking with them, she had gleaned other perspectives, fresh views that moved her in her thinking about perceived failures in the past. She was affirmed in her identity as a loving parent and partner and was looking forward to becoming a grandparent again, as one of her sons was having a child of his own. With the prospect of new life beginning, this circle of life instilled hope that the intergenerational pattern of abuse and silence over what had happened would not be replicated in the next generation.

Lastly, women survivors of CSA need to begin to understand the limitations they have encountered in their family of origin in relation to changing ageing parents' attitudes about the original CSA. This is important if survivors were disbelieved or the sexual abuse was minimised by authority figures within the family when they were growing up as a child or adolescent. In these situations, as adults, they may need to consider setting limits and boundaries for their own well-being in terms of revisiting the past abuse if the reaction is likely to be negative again. In the case of parents who are dementing or mentally unable to empathise owing to cognitive decline, survivors' attempts or further attempts may trigger another experience of not being heard or understood. Ideally, discussing disclosure or re-disclosure to ageing perpetrators or family members should be prepared for in therapy to assess whether or how to disclose in these circumstances. The emotional engagement of an elderly non-offending parent in having a conversation about earlier abuse may not be possible for a host of reasons. However, the loss of a relationship with the perpetrator(s) and, in some cases, entire families of origin can be grieved. The difficulties of parenting and of behaving in ways that likely impacted the next generation can also be lamented and perhaps laid to rest to some extent.

In the next chapter, the impact of the global COVID-19 pandemic as a major historical event will be reflected on in relation to the kinds of challenges it brought for women survivors and their disclosure of CSA.

References

Alaggia, R., Collin-Vezina, D., & Lateef, R. (2019). Facilitators and barriers to child sexual abuse (CSA) disclosures: a research update (2000–2016). *Trauma, Violence, and Abuse*, 20(2), 260–283. doi:10.1177/1524838017697312

Brazelton, J. (2011). African American women looking back: making meaning of the disclosure process of incest survivors across the life course. *Dissertation Abstracts International: Section A. Humanities and Social Sciences*, 72(2-A), 738.

Brazelton, J. F. (2015). The secret storm: exploring the disclosure process of African American women survivors of child sexual abuse across the life course. *Traumatology*, 21(3), 181.

Burgess, A. W., & Phillips, S. L. (2006). Sexual abuse, trauma and dementia in the elderly: a retrospective study of 284 cases. *Victims & Offenders*, 1(2), 193–204. doi:10.1080/15564880600663935

Gibson, K., Morgan., M., Woolley, C., & Powis, T. (2011). Growing up at Centrepoint: retrospective accounts of childhood spent at an intentional community. *Journal of Child Sexual Abuse*, 20(4), 413–434. doi:10.1080/10538712.2011.591364

Graham, K., Patterson, T., Justice, T., & Rapsey, C. (2022). 'It's not a great boulder, it's just a piece of baggage': older women's reflections on healing from childhood sexual abuse. *Journal of Interpersonal Violence*, 37(1–2),705–725.

Halvorsen, J. E., Solberg, E. T., & Stige, S. H. (2020). 'To say it out loud is to kill your own childhood.' – An exploration of the first person perspective of barriers to disclosing child sexual abuse. *Children and Youth Services Review*, 113. doi:10.1016/j.childyouth.2020.104999

Lee, C., Tsenkova, V., & Carr, D. (2014). Childhood trauma and metabolic syndrome in men and women. *Social Science & Medicine*, 105, 122–130.

Leibrich, J. (2015). *Sanctuary: The Discovery of Wonder*. Otago University Press.

McElvaney, R. (2015). Disclosure of child sexual abuse: delays, non-disclosure and partial disclosure. What the research tells us and implications for practice. *Child Abuse Review*, 24(3), 159–169. doi:10.1002/car.2280

McGregor, K., Julich, S., Glover, M., & Gautam, J. (2010). Health professionals' responses to disclosure of child sexual abuse history: female child sexual abuse survivors' experiences. *Journal of Child Sexual Abuse*, 19(3), 239–254. doi:10.1080/10538711003789015

Monahan, K. (2010). Themes of adult sibling sexual abuse survivors in later life: an initial exploration. *Clinical Social Work Journal*, 38, 361–369.

Mooney, J. L., & McGregor, C. (2018). How adults tell: messages for society and policy makers regarding disclosures of childhood sexual abuse. Unpublished PhD thesis. School of Political Science and Sociology, National University of Ireland, Galway.

Pack, M. (2002). Sexual abuse counsellors' responses to stress and trauma: a social work perspective. Unpublished PhD thesis, Victoria University of Wellington, New Zealand.

Pack, M. (2010). Career themes in the lives of sexual abuse counsellors. *New Zealand Journal of Counselling*, 30(2), 75–92.

Rajan, G., Wahlstrom, L., Philips, B., Wandell, P., Wachtler, C., Svedin, C. G., & Carlsson, A. C. (2021). Delayed healthcare access among victims of sexual abuse, understood through internal and external gatekeeping mechanisms. *Nordic Journal of Psychiatry*, 75(5), 370–377. doi:10.1080/08039488.2020.1868573

Sorsoli, L. (2010). 'I remember', 'I thought', 'I know I didn't say': silence and memory in trauma narratives. *Memory*, 18(2), 129–141.

Wager, N. M. (2013). Sexual revictimization: double betrayal and the risk associated with dissociative amnesia. *Journal of Child Sexual Abuse*, 22(7), 878–899. doi:10.1080/10538712.2013.830666

Walbridge, J. (2021). Telling the truth to oneself, listening to the truths of others. *Psychoanalysis Self and Context*, 16(2), 126–129. doi:10.1080/24720038.2021.1892694

White, M. (1995). *Re-authoring Lives: Interviews and Essays*. Adelaide, South Australia: Dulwich Centre.

7 The disclosure of CSA by women survivors in the context of the global pandemic of COVID-19

> Our team of mental health clinicians has not been immune to the far-reaching impacts of the pandemic, personally and professionally. Through the first wave of the Covid-19 outbreak we were all primarily working from our homes while adjusting to the abrupt transition to virtual mental health care. Despite some initial reservations, we adapted fairly quickly to the technical components, learned to be less flustered by glitches that were bound to happen, and had back up plans in place in the event of disconnection.
>
> (Ontario, Canada-based clinicians reflect on their experiences of adapting their outpatient therapy service to the new environment of the global pandemic; Azzopardi et al., 2022, pp. 9–10)

Introduction

This chapter explores the impact of the COVID-19 pandemic on disclosure for women survivors of CSA. The global pandemic of COVID-19 has been described as a 'traumatic event' that involves 'a potential threat to self and close others' survival' (Tsur & Abu-Raiya, 2020, p. 10). More generally, researchers have found that the pandemic saw a rise in severe grief responses at a societal level as we grieved the demise of a proportion of our population across borders (*New Scientist*, 2020). Women survivors of CSA may have lost loved ones to the virus and may have lost their jobs linked to social networks and identities during the years pre- and post-COVID-19. The social structure of our society was reorganised owing to restrictions imposed by national governments around the globe. Gatherings of people for celebrations such as weddings and christenings and commemorations such as memorials and funerals were limited during lockdown restrictions, and communal events and gatherings were postponed. When we are required to social distance and to phone, email or text rather than come in person, grief can develop around the lack of face-to-face contact. Sometimes, during restrictions, the lack of face-to-face contact could happen suddenly and be prolonged for weeks and even months (*New Scientist*, 2020, p. 8).

Survivor guilt in families who lost some family members through death from post-COVID-19 complications while others survived, the inability to say

DOI: 10.4324/9781032669205-7

farewell to loved ones in hospitals or rest homes, and new protocols in hospitals for visiting inpatients meant that people may have lacked opportunities to reach out to others and to dying relatives. In the post-COVID-19 environment, they may still be healing from such events. With these kinds of heightened grief and loss responses, memories and flashbacks of CSA can become prominent again for women survivors of CSA. With the economic recession that was an outcome of the global restrictions to curb the spread of the virus, the potential for various forms of family violence has been identified (Usher et al., 2020). Specifically, domestic violence, including child maltreatment, has been found to increase at this time (van Berkel et al., 2020). The heightened need for services has been hampered by the lack of availability of meaningful options for support, however (Usher et al., 2020). Given these issues and the likelihood they would colour the environment in which women disclose historical CSA, a literature review focused on the impact of the COVID-19 pandemic was undertaken. The description of the search strategy and the results are reported in the following:

Search strategy and results of literature search on the topic

I undertook a subsequent search on women's experience of sexual abuse, historical CSA disclosure and domestic violence during lockdown conditions. The following databases were searched:

- Medline
- Ebsco including CINAHL
- Scopus
- PsycINFO
- Proquest
- PubMed
- LitCovid
- Factiva
- Google

Both academic journals and media were searched for the topics mentioned above. News media coverage reported women's anecdotal experiences of lockdown during the Covid-19 Pandemic and so media sources were included in the expanded search parameters. The academic literature was more theoretical than qualitative. In future, there will likely be more academic research on the topic owing to the recent and current nature of the topic. Unfortunately, I was unable to find many relevant results on the issue of disclosure of CSA in the context of the global COVID-19 pandemic specifically. I found only six results initially, which reflects the newness of the topic and the fact that researchers were in a situation of self-isolation as they conducted the studies. To widen the search and potentially increase the number of hits in electronic databases of the international peer-reviewed research literature, I later expanded the search strategy to find anything relating to sexual abuse disclosure and teleconsultations, but that didn't help very much. I also searched for 'historical sexual abuse' and 'COVID-19', without the 'disclosure' concept, but still found very little on the topic. I searched Medline, PsycINFO, PubMed, Scopus and Google Scholar with these key words. In the print media, there were some examples of women survivors who tried but failed to get their needs met, with the restrictions making access to care (whether medical or counselling) far more difficult than in non-COVID-19 times. I decided to include these examples in the search.

Themes from the literature

The themes of the literature review that follows are:

1. The increasing incidence of various kinds of interlocking abuse (domestic violence, child abuse and maltreatment) with the declining availability of service options for medical and therapeutic help and the formal reporting of CSA
2. The ill health and death of significant others, including the perpetrator of CSA and other elderly family members. Their deaths had the effect of reigniting memories of CSA without the usual ceremonies of funeral and family gatherings as an opportunity to grieve communally
3. Periods of lockdown restrictions leading to greater social isolation for those women survivors of CSA whose main social contact was predominantly at work, in personal therapy or in community/group settings. I have hypothesised this isolation as intensifying the 'shame–self-stigmatisation' spiral mentioned in the previous chapters of this book. Without the safe haven of relationships to support the survivors' ongoing need for disclosure and retelling of their CSA
4. The cultural norms of some ethnic groups are challenged by not having access to face-to-face interaction; acknowledgement of the physical and spiritual health needs being connected, and the right to communal rituals and ceremonies were highlighted. The example of Makere deals with holistic care and, specifically, Māori health and well-being principles that are recommended in Aotearoa New Zealand under the Treaty of Waitangi regarding responsibilities in health care. These principles are discussed in the context of changes in health care that occurred during the pandemic

We will now explore each of the themes highlighted from this literature search in the sections below.

The effects of the global COVID-19 pandemic on family violence and the availability of helping services

For those women who were living in situations of lockdown restrictions, domestic violence was found to feature more prominently than previously. Violence against women during the pandemic restrictions has been documented internationally (Roesch et al., 2020). Increased incidence of domestic violence against women was a feature of the stay-at-home orders in many countries (Kofman et al., 2020). As women survivors are often found to select partners who go on to abuse them, reminding them of their original childhood abuse, feelings of history repeating itself and the helplessness/hopelessness spiral can mean that the home becomes a dangerous context, when normally this might be seen as a safe haven or sanctuary. This has led some researchers to see the home during periods of quarantine as being a hotbed of agitation and frustration, fuelling acts of domestic violence (Mazza et al., 2020). The assessment of domestic violence across domains of functioning with a multidisciplinary approach is seen as being the most effective approach in these circumstances, with psychological, physical and emotional domains being assessed by a team of psychiatrists, social workers, psychologists and refuge and legal personnel (Mazza et al., 2020).

Obtaining the support needed to leave the situation is a theme of this literature. Support from helping and significant others is still outlined as one of the major protective factors discussed in the literature, enabling the woman to rebound and to build a new life (Wright et al., 2022). However, help to get out of an abusive situation was less immediately available during the lockdown restrictions. Many of the advocacy services in the United States shifted face-to-face services to telehealth during the pandemic. One such project was the Pennsylvania Coalition Against Rape (PCAR), which reported how a change in access affected the utilisation of its services during the initial COVID-19 restrictions between 2019 and 2020. The evaluation discovered that there was a 37% drop in telephone calls to their helpline from March to April 2020, when restrictions commenced. The helpline's number of calls increased when restrictions were easing in June 2020, with a 34% increase (Wright et al., 2022). When 2019 figures were compared to those for 2020, the number of calls for advocacy was still 31% lower. The authors account for the decrease in the utilisation of the helpline for domestic abuse being related to the obstacles posed to effective help seeking during the COVID-19 restrictions. Periods of lockdown made it difficult to access help acutely, and advocacy services were virtually unavailable. In particular, the worry of leaving home to travel to the centre to discuss financial issues or health problems and loss of childcare were considered to be factors in the reduction of numbers calling the helpline (Wright et al., 2022). When locked down with an abuser, it may have been impossible for a woman to have enough personal space to make a confidential phone call. In these situations, the authors advocate for developing a safety plan with the survivor on how to identify the most appropriate mode of contact and timing of the contact; educating the survivor to store helpline numbers under names that are not identifiable as helplines; and identifying a trusted friend or family member to be a mediator between the survivor and advocates' or counsellors' calls (Wright et al., 2022).

Family disconnection, illness of family members, loss and grieving

When issues relating to sexual abuse from the past were reignited through the death of the perpetrator of the abuse, or the non-offending caregiver died, the need to revisit the memories of the past and also current issues might be delayed until a time when there could be face-to-face contact with a counsellor. If the counselling facility was located in a hospital, there could be fears of a higher risk of exposure to the virus, particularly if the survivor had compromised general health, long-term health issues such as respiratory conditions or was in the 60+ age group with predisposing risk factors for long-term negative health outcomes if they contracted the virus.

More men than women died from COVID-19, suggesting that women were more often caregivers through this time, increasing both their exposure to the virus and emotional exhaustion from prolonged periods of caregiving (Gausman & Langer, 2020; Wright et al., 2022).

Social isolation during lockdowns

During lockdowns and when social isolation is mandated, there is evidence that this disconnection from interacting with supportive others exacerbates the experience of shame in the disclosure of CSA. Shame is more likely in these kinds of conditions, as the lack of potential for meaningful interaction turns reflection on one's abuse inward, galvanising the inner critic. Partly this has been linked to longer periods of social isolation exposing underlying pre-existing and new vulnerabilities. The length of lockdown periods or recurrent periods of lockdown with little warning increase the risks of negative mental health outcomes in the community (van Gelder et al., 2020). The lack of ease of access to the protective factors of connection, through attachment and support, heightens the vulnerabilities of individuals, families and their local communities (Usher et al., 2020).

Compounding these vulnerabilities, shame, self-blame and self-stigmatisation for being a victim of CSA have been discovered to be predictors of revictimisation in current intimate relationships (MacGinley et al., 2019, pp. 1141–1142). These authors posit that the shame internalised by the survivor develops in a socio-cultural context. The survivor's internalised shame continues in a spiralling fashion, without any social connection to enable disclosure (MacGinley et al., 2019, pp. 1141–1142).

Social disconnection was experienced by whole populations during the periods of lockdown and associated closures of social support agencies due to social sanctions preventing face-to-face contact. In such a social context as a global pandemic, this sense of shame can potentially engulf the self completely. If there are insufficient buffering or protective factors present, as outlined in previous chapters, consequences such as self-blame and avoidance, which in earlier chapters I have referred to as the self-stigmatisation spiral, can re-emerge.

Different types of telling

Summarising earlier chapters, there are different ways in which adult women survivors tell of their historical CSA. These types of disclosure are not mutually exclusive, and women may choose several kinds of disclosure throughout the life course, with telling being an iterative, discursive process. These types are summarised, with the originating authors, in the following:

- 'First tellings' (Gasker, 1999): this is the first time historical CSA is discussed with anyone else. Gasker discusses the first time telling of adult women survivors she has worked with in her clinical practice. First tellings involve a true leap of faith as they rely on how accurately the woman has gauged the safety of the confident and the relationship in which to tell
- 'Indirect telling' (Alaggia & Kirshenbaum, 2005) refers to when a woman survivor chooses not to disclose but becomes suddenly upset and/or cannot deal with the tension of not being able to tell. She may say what happened in a symbolic acting out, or it might be enacted behaviourally in some way. Some behaviours can, therefore, be seen as a type of symbolic disclosure, such as cutting behaviours to alleviate internally generated shame or stress related to CSA. The survivor cannot verbally or openly express herself owing to the nature of the trauma, with the tendency towards dissociation
- 'Partial telling' (Alaggia & Kirshenbaum, 2005): this mode of disclosure involves some aspects of the CSA being disclosed and others not, drawing from the survivor's understanding of what is safe to tell
- 'Formal telling' and 'informal telling' (Alaggia & Kirshenbaum, 2005): informal telling is where the survivor tells family and informal supporters such as friends or partners. Formal telling usually involves reports made via legal representatives, police or child protection authorities, or other bodies such as royal commissions that seek legal action and redress through policy and organisational change
- 'Immediate telling' or 'direct telling' (McElvaney et al., 2014): this type of telling is when the survivor tells another of the CSA prompted by direct questioning by others, including teachers, peers, friends, partners and others who may notice a change in behaviour and ask the survivor, 'what's wrong?' This is particularly a feature of adolescent tellings about CSA
- 'Delayed telling' (McElvaney, 2015): this mode of telling, both informally to family and friends and more formally to authorities (child protection services, police, legal representatives), is paused for a period of time as the conditions may not be considered 'safe' or the confident deemed to be the right person to whom to disclose. Shame may also be operating to delay disclosure
- 'Pressure cooker-inspired immediate telling' or 'unintentional telling' (McElvaney et al., 2014; McElvaney, 2015): this model of telling was developed by McElvaney as a dynamic underlying many disclosures of CSA. A triggering event or feeling might suddenly lead to a disclosure or

not, as it could result in an immediate or indirect telling, as detailed above. The 'pressure cooker effect' reflects the survivor's conflict of wanting to tell but also wanting to keep her abuse secret and undisclosed. The pressure of these conflicting tensions pulling in different directions may produce a sudden and unintended disclosure of CSA

- Telling that is made then retracted: in this scenario, the woman survivor tells owing to the pressure cooker effect or as an immediate telling but then withdraws her disclosure for a variety of reasons. A disclosure followed by retraction is often seen owing to family mores, cultural beliefs against disclosure due to loyalty to family or the subordinate status of women in society
- No telling or non-disclosure of CSA

Types of telling during the pandemic

Women who disclosed historical CSA were thought to be more often triggered to tell the story of their CSA at this time of global fear, with its associated loss of community and connection to others. For example, some theorists suggested that the threat of catching the virus could trigger feelings associated with child sexual abuse as people could not easily control whether they picked up the virus and became unwell. The feeling of being abused by the felt powerlessness of the situation could trigger issues related to historical CSA. Second, the longer-term health impacts of long COVID, once contracted, may have a long health and well-being legacy, like child sexual abuse (Roesch et al., 2020).

The under-reporting of child maltreatment and domestic violence during COVID-19 is now well documented. The stress of not being able to disclose was exacerbated by the closure of services, difficulties reaching out when the perpetrator was locked down with the victim, job loss, social isolation and collective grief due to bereavement on a community and societal level. In this situation, there can be more immediate tellings or those made because of the 'pressure cooker effect' (McElvaney et al., 2014, p. 93).

The mandate to be immunised against COVID-19 similarly could be particularly triggering for CSA survivors as, again, self-determination, choice and autonomy may seem to be compromised or infringed in the interests of protecting others and the wider community. A recent study of CSA survivors' distress throughout the peak stages of the COVID-19 pandemic between March and May 2020, when Israel was in a situation of total lockdown, discovered that the CSA participants showed a heightened sense of distress compared to those in a sample of adults without a CSA history (Tsur & Abu-Raiya, 2020). The fear of COVID-19 was assessed using a five-point Likert scale linked to questions about the impact of COVID-19 on the individual. While both male and female survivors were included in the CSA sample, women reported higher rates of distress during the national lockdown in Israel. Those CSA survivors who were women were found more likely to have a single or divorced relationship status, which may also be seen as a legacy of their abuse (Tsur & Abu-Raiya, 2020). Those reporting a history of CSA were also more likely to earn less income and so be more economically deprived. The authors conclude that it was not the fact that individuals had a history of trauma that meant they were more likely to have a heightened experience of distress during periods of lockdown, but it was rather related to the fact they were still actively dealing with the after-effects and sequelae of CSA in the present in situations of social isolation. The finding that many women survivors of CSA were also living alone, as their relationship status was more often single or divorced, meant that isolation might have kept the cycle of traumatisation mentioned in previous chapters active in their experience of day-to-day life. In such extreme situations, there may be no one with whom to process issues related to the aftermath of CSA as they arise under the restrictions of lockdown. While COVID-19 may not have a direct causal relationship to this distress, the isolation and difficulties in disclosing one's experience day to day likely confounded the overall healing journey for women survivors whose usual social interaction was limited or not possible in a situation of quarantine or isolation.

The emergence of the COVID-19 global health pandemic and the economic impact of governmental restrictions placed on individuals and their families introduced, for many survivors and their supporters, multiple interlocking obstacles to both disclosure and getting the care needed. Practically, the therapeutic relationship, which historically had relied on face-to-face contact in an agency or office setting, became less possible during successive government lockdowns, and so health providers needed to make a paradigm shift to online and virtual contexts during those unprecedented times to provide opportunities for disclosing historical abuse and trauma. Periods of recurring lockdown, daily mask use and physical distancing measures necessitated an abrupt transition from traditional in-person health care to virtual telemedicine using Zoom, videoconferencing, Skype-type technologies or cell phones. While, for some women, the pandemic meant a time of new and exciting opportunities using these new platforms for communication, this shift is not without challenges. In the emerging literature on the aftermath of COVID-19, exploring the lessons to be learned, it is acknowledged that there were unique implications for practising as a health care professional at that time. Trauma-informed interventions based on the health care professional's knowledge and experience still needed to offer the safe context and relationship in which survivors could feel supported enough to raise historical issues relating to earlier experiences of sexual abuse.

An illustration of the shame–self-stigmatisation spiral: Jessie's and Makere's case studies

Attributing blame to oneself for one's experiences of CSA has longer-term consequences for help seeking by women survivors of CSA. Finding opportunities for connection and disclosure of both CSA and the after-effects became more problematic during the global pandemic. The narratives of women survivors who were going through struggles with such issues during the COVID-19 pandemic are summarized in the narratives based on two composite case studies I will refer to as Jessie and Makere.

Background to the case studies

During the national lockdown of March 2020 in Aotearoa New Zealand due to the global threat of the COVID-19 virus, two women of differing ages, one 22 and the other 49, tried to get help for the physical problems they were experiencing as a result of early childhood sexual abuse, in a women's health clinic. During the COVID-19 pandemic in New Zealand, this clinic was inundated with women who presented with concerns about the impact of the virus on their general health. Both Makere and Jessie were attempting to get their claims for sexual abuse accepted by the ACC (Accident Compensation and Rehabilitation Corporation), the statutory authority dealing with sensitive claims. They were seeking assistance with differing medical problems that had been diagnosed in the hospital and related to the ongoing legacy of their original sexual abuse.

Although, prior to the pandemic, they had been examined, diagnosed and treated in face-to-face mode in the hospital context, where patients continued to be seen in this mode, staff in most other government departments were working remotely by freephone and email from home offices. The women's different cultural backgrounds influenced what they needed for their recovery in terms of services and treatment, and both struggled to have their physical issues, influenced by a history of CSA, acknowledged by the health and compensation authorities during lockdown.

The tendency for the medical model to focus attention on physical health by separating cultural well-being from spiritual and psychological well-being is a recurring theme in both case studies. In the residual model of health offered by a public health system, the part of the body with the diagnosed problem is usually treated. This model contrasts with the notion of well-being in more holistic models, such as those developed within a Māori-centred model of health and well-being. In their literature review of the indigenous Māori models of health, the authors of one study highlighted the importance of relational approaches to engaging Māori and their *whānau*, or extended family networks (Wilson et al., 2021). There are three guiding principles for working with Māori in the health care system from these authors' perspective, which involve *whakawhanaungatanga, manaakitanga* and *wairua*. First, using concepts of *whakawhanaungatanga* is considered to be the first guiding principle of a holistic health care model. *Whakawhanaungatanga* relates to the process of establishing relationships using culturally specific protocols and informed by values of *aroha*, or compassion. *Manaakitanga* is the second guiding principle for working with Māori and involves providing hospitality and kindness, *mauri*, or fellowship by bringing people together. Third, the dimension of *wāirua*, or spirituality, is central to our understanding of health from a bicultural perspective (Wilson et al., 2021). It is my experience in evaluating health services for Pacific peoples that hospitality extends to assisting with transport to treatment, welcoming the client in the reception area and offering tea and coffee and providing a choice of worker, by gender and culture, from workers who can speak in the client's language. Confidentiality is especially important when dealing with matters of the body, such as sexual health and gynaecology. For women survivors who have had their bodily boundaries violated in childhood, sensitivity when dealing with the areas of the body that are considered to be *tapu*, or sacred, is considered essential. These are often the parts of the body involved in reproduction, as they are seen as being the crucible of life. The restrictions enforced by COVID-19 often worked against the practitioners who were endeavouring to work from these central principles or in these ways, seen as being biculturally responsive, as the following case studies illustrate.

Jessie's story

Jessie is a 22-year-old professional athlete of Pākehā (European of New Zealand) descent who, over the years of her professional career, had had a variety of injuries from her sport and came to the hospital with severe chronic pelvic pain that was unrelated to any previous physical injury. She had spent five years struggling with this pain of unknown origin when her general practitioner referred her to the women's gynaecological service for investigation of its causes. After investigative surgery for endometriosis, where nothing was found but polycystic ovary symptoms were noted, she saw a gynaecologist to whom she disclosed a combination of pain during penetrative sex and involuntary muscle spasms known as vaginismus. Her gynaecologist diagnosed that she had a condition known as genitopelvic pain. The gynaecologist advised her that the treatment for this condition is usually pelvic physiotherapy in combination with psychological interventions and relaxation training. As the doctor did follow-up by a telephone call, with telemedicine being the norm in the hospital in the early months of the pandemic, Jessie never disclosed that she had a sensitive claim for sexual abuse events when she was 14 years old. As her claim was for psychological intervention for mental trauma, she asked her case manager if she could be referred to a pelvic physiotherapist, and this request was declined as she was advised by the national compensation and rehabilitation agency in New Zealand (ACC) that there are no such physical treatments covered by a claim for mental injury. She did continue to have sessions with a counsellor for her sexual abuse recovery on Skype, but these were less frequent during the lockdown conditions. Her counsellor for her CSA connected the recent physical-genitopelvic pain diagnosis with the psychological legacy of her sexual abuse. Her therapist suggested that she return to her general practitioner to lodge a further claim for physical injury for the sexual abuse events as there was no integrated body therapy covered under her sensitive claim for mental injury.

Jessie again was seen by the general practitioner via telemedicine, on Zoom, as physical examinations were not possible at this point in the COVID-19 restrictions. The general practitioner accepted Jessie's request to lodge a physical compensation claim based on the earlier report she had on file from the gynaecologist. Her general practitioner was aware that a further claim for physical rehabilitation under a physical injury claim would provide the appropriate treatment for her diagnosis.

This application for a claim for cover of a physical injury was declined by the ACC, and she was referred back to her counsellor for continuing psychosocial support and counselling. During lockdown, her counsellor continued with sessions on Skype, noting that, whenever Jessie had an altercation on the phone with her case manager or general practitioner, she both became disheartened and started blaming herself. It was around this time that Jessie became distressed by the decline decision on her physical rehabilitation and, out of desperation, returned to cutting her arms as a way of physically expressing her frustration. It was a combination of feeling unheard and of not being validated as having a physical injury linked to historical abuse that tipped the balance. Jessie had difficulties with communicating and found remote technologies to be the most difficult to communicate with. The act of self-harming and avoidance kept the self-stigmatisation–shame spiral going. She began re-experiencing the guilt she had felt at not being able to stop her abuse as an adolescent. She was living on her own and supporting herself on sickness benefit, which further played into her sense of frustration and of being misunderstood.

Finally, at the conclusion of lockdown and with her counsellor advocating for her, her physical pain was accepted as being part of her mental injury by her ACC case manager, then a year after diagnosis. With the opening-up of services for face-to-face contact, Jessie was to see a pelvic physiotherapist. Unfortunately, the region locked down again, leading to delays in her being seen by the physiotherapist.

These delays in being seen in person by health professionals retriggered feelings associated with her original abuse in that she felt re-victimised and powerless to obtain the help she needed. The lockdown periods, with access to health care and government agencies only through distance and remote technologies, drove Jessie further down 'the shame spiral'.

This case illustrates how the compartmentalisation of the body into physical and psychological aspects can miss the interrelationship between mind and body, which is a theme for many adult women who have conditions that are both physical and psychological in nature. Many physical pain conditions have their origins in a history of CSA. Having been raised in a family where she could not openly discuss her abuse, she edited these recollections of her CSA out of her narrative until physical pain made her think about seeking help. Working with different systems – the public compensation scheme for sexual abuse, the hospital specialist, her general practitioner and the physiotherapist – to gain help for her pain was impeded by the lack of co-ordination between the various governmental agencies involved. They each attended to their specialism while not understanding the holistic way that CSA, through the symptomology of pain, was impacting her relationships and her life. Having to navigate complex bureaucratic systems during a time when face-to-face contact was impossible compounded the dilemma, and, had it not been for the advocacy of the ongoing relationship with her therapist, Jessie could have easily given up, with her needs falling into the cracks between parts of a system that did not communicate well together.

In a similar but different narrative, we connect with Makere and her story of obtaining holistic and culturally responsive health care during the historically difficult time of the COVID-19 pandemic.

Makere's story

The second case study is of Makere, a 49-year-old woman of Māori descent and culture, who lives with extended family on a local *marae*, or meeting place/community. Makere has suffered intermittently from reduced immune function, chronic fatigue and muscle pain throughout her life. More recently, she has felt that her health problems are linked to her sexual abuse, between the ages of five and seven, at the hands of a relative during times spend on the *marae* with extended *whānau* (family). Because of the discovery of a large mass that tested as being cancerous, she opted to have a hysterectomy (removal of the uterus) at the age of 24 years. Many years after her hysterectomy, she began connecting her early abuse to her early diagnosis of cervical cancer with its links to the HPV virus, which is associated with sexual health and past sexual partners. She was aware that she had struggled physically with health issues in her teenage years and commented that she felt shame and self-loathing as a young person. As a soon-to-be 50 year old, she believed that the guilt and shame had gone to her most sacred place, her uterus, considered *tapu* by Māori owing to the womb's association with child bearing and life-giving potential. Owing to her deep sense of shame, she had never told anyone about her abuse until she was approaching her 50s. She commented that she felt that she was living in a 'traumatised body', even though her abuse occurred during childhood and her cancer diagnosis and treatment were when she was in her 20s. Both were now in the past. She had not been able to have children after the hysterectomy and often felt resentful and 'ripped off' for not being able to fulfil this potential to have a family. These connections in different parts of her life narrative and parts of her body coalesced in her thinking and became heightened as issues arose during the global pandemic. She said it was the time of global grief and suffering that, for her, 'connected the dots' to her own abuse and subsequent health issues. Interestingly, it was in this time of global suffering that she felt less alone with her own pain from the various sources of grief she experienced as a consequence of her early abuse.

'Connecting the dots'

This experience of 'connecting the dots' during a period of lockdown echoes Tsur and Abu-Raiya's findings in the Israeli context that issues related to the sequelae of child sexual abuse may be highlighted or compounded during a period of COVID-19 restriction (Tsur & Abu- Raiya, 2020). Makere sought help from the publicly funded rehabilitation unit dealing with sexual abuse claims and contacted a national call centre through a national freephone she found online. No face-to-face contact would have been possible owing to the restrictions imposed nationally by a level-4 lockdown. A call centre operator said she would leave a message with an assessor who would telephone her back in due course. The psychologist who contacted her diagnosed in a tele-consultation a range of mental health issues affecting her currently, including PTSD, chronic depressive disorder and generalised anxiety involving panic attacks. The psychologist sent a referral for an occupational therapist to visit on the lifting of some of the COVID-19 restrictions so that they could meet face-to-face, with mask wearing and social distancing, in Makere's home. Owing to the restrictions, it took a month to get to the actual assessment, which looked at how the abuse had impacted her life in a number of key areas. She was notified of the result of this assessment by letter two weeks after her in-person assessment. This letter informed her that the assessor had assessed a 20% impairment rating, which meant she was eligible for a small allowance each month. Makere felt a 20% impairment rating for mental injury related to her history of CSA did not accurately reflect the damage she had sustained, and she knew she had the right to appeal this decision so that it could be reviewed by an impartial mediation service and the right to appoint a legal advocate or representative to defend her at the hearing. However, she did not wish to go through another prolonged period of applying for an assessment and waiting for the assessor, to go through exactly the same process again. The assessment consumed several days of her time as she prepared herself to discuss personal details with a complete stranger coming to her home in an emotionally intense and difficult process. She wondered if it would be worth being reassessed as she was shocked that, after going through the whole process, involving remote and in-person interviews, the impact of the mental injury in monetary terms was worth so little.

The assessment aimed to consider the mental injury inflicted on the client's life subsequently. This includes activities of daily living, social functioning, concentration, persistence and pace, and adaptation/decompensation. The assessment represented her functioning as a snapshot in time, with the underlying expectations that the client would wish to seek counselling with the aim of improving the rating assessed over time. However, Makere did not wish to seek therapy in the traditional western modes offered, preferring to process her feelings within her culture, drawing upon the help of spiritual healers (*tohunga*). As an adult, she felt spiritually tarnished by her experience of CSA and violated on a 'soul level'. She had a strong intuition that this kind of spiritual healing would not be publicly available as a funded service through ACC, and especially not during a national pandemic.

Makere forged her own pathway to healing from CSA by asking for spiritual healing offered within a Māori framework for recovery of her health and well-being. The process of home visits from the occupational therapist was problematic for Makere as she lived in a community settlement close to the *marae*, or meeting house. Finding a confidential space was often difficult for this reason.

It took a further six months to have 24 sessions approved, with a Māori healer using an approach that drew from a Rongoā Māori framework (a form of holistic healing indigenous to Māori involving mind–body–spiritual dimensions of health). At first, she was advised that the provider would only offer *Mirimiri* or traditional body work/massage or *karakia* (prayer) or cultural support and advice. Spiritual healing may encompass aspects of all these individual therapies, but they need to be comprehensively offered in face-to-face mode to respond to Makere's particular issues. However, re-requesting traditional healing through telephone calls to her case manager meant that her persistence paid off, and Makere was eventually offered the funded holistic spiritual healing she had requested from the government rehabilitation agency.

After 24 individual sessions, she found that her life had been transformed by this form of spiritual healing. Visual flashbacks of her abuse lessened owing to management of the physical symptoms of the 'fight or flight' response that would be triggered by the shame spiral she experienced. Breaking the fight or flight cycle in the body and mind, she felt, was bringing her into a better state of health. She believes conventional therapies do not work for her, or for many women survivors, as the body therapies need to be longer term. Those physiotherapy sessions that are bounded by time or number of sessions tend to be very short term. Longer-term body and cultural therapies are often considered too expensive by some public funding bodies and, during the COVID-19 restrictions, may have been completely unavailable as the *Rongoā*, or traditional healing system, involves the use of plant-based remedies tailored to the needs of the individual. *Rongoā* is about the well-being of the individual and the *whenua* (land) and the waters that flow over the land. Similarly, *Mirimiri*, which may be offered as part of *Rongoā*, is a traditional form of physical bodywork and massage that has spiritual aspects such as *karakia*, or prayer, incorporated as part of the body therapy. All of these approaches, which are relational, need to be offered in face-to-face mode.

Working remotely and the potential for re-traumatisation

Although the benefits of remote counselling and recovery work through Skype-type technologies are acknowledged in the research reviewed, there are also some difficulties documented around technology literacy, cultural factors and the fact some trauma survivors have great difficulty connecting without the person being physically in the room (Butler et al., 2023, p. 7). Some practitioners report that they are needing to enquire about the details of the abuse, and this relies on the survivor thinking about and recalling the original trauma. It is difficult to gauge the impact of retelling remotely, on-screen, using Skype-type platforms for communication. Conversely, some found that, during COVID-19 lockdown restrictions, clients who usually missed their appointments did attend virtually. Practitioners interviewed for one Australian study said that clients would attend from the comfort of their own homes, whereas normally they would miss an appointment to come into the office. It seemed that Zoom calling from home was supportive to their coping strategies as they could talk from their home where they felt safe and yet separated from the practitioner (Butler et al., 2023).

One agency in the Canadian context developed a teleconsultation service using an ecological systems lens to deliver therapy through online platforms (Azzopardi et al., 2022). In Ontario, where the authors were practising, all non-essential workplaces closed, and a state of emergency was declared, thwarting the efforts to reach survivors of CSA to reduce the risk of further psychological harm. Aware of these obstacles, the agency implemented a multidisciplinary team meeting to plan for the likely impacts for clients and their families. The outpatient side of their service embraced the various online platforms for delivering therapy with a view to ensuring practitioner well-being as they offered services from the office and from home. Extra attention was given to the multifaceted nature of CSA trauma compounded by distress evoked by the day-to-day experience of the pandemic, with suicidality being closely assessed by 'systematic screening' that involved an agreed assessment tool (Azzopardi et al., 2022, p. 8).

An example of a case shared with the mental health services during the 2020 lockdown in New Zealand illustrates how difficult it was for survivors locked down in a 'bubble' when the family context turned out to be a 'bubble of trouble'.

Mai's story

Mai was a 15 year old, also known by her Middle Eastern name that means 'quiet' or 'peaceful' in her language. She came into the emergency department where she was triaged by the on-call crisis resolution mental health team. Her parents accompanied her as she was hearing voices or auditory hallucinations. She recounted that she had noted that the television had been sending her messages saying that she was a 'bad girl' for not doing what her father had asked her to do. Another voice said that she had brought shame on her family by not getting a good report from her school for her academic work. Once assessed, she was admitted to hospital as an inpatient because of persistent suicidal ideation. She told the assessing psychologist that she wished to cut her wrists to make the voices 'go away'. Her parents looked very concerned for her safety, and a younger sister and older brother were accompanied by their parents.

The ward nurses noted that she would say she 'hated' her father when asked about how things were at home. She said she was writing a letter to let him know this, but each time she wrote she would tear up the page and put it in the rubbish bin. When her clinical psychologist asked what her anger at her father was about, she finally disclosed inappropriate touching from school age, usually at night or when her mother was out of the house. The auditory hallucinations developed when her father was home from work during a month-long lockdown, at which time she felt more at risk from his inappropriate touching. She had tried to tell her mother about the abuse at this time, but she said Mai must forgive any wrongdoing by her father who was head of their household. Furthermore, she must say nothing further to avoid bringing shame on herself and the family. Her mother told Mai it would split the family up if she told anyone, and her sister and brother would be without their father if he was prosecuted. Her mother arrived at Mai's bedside begging her 'not to tell' and crying daily, as she did not wish her husband's behaviour to be reported to the authorities. Once Mai had disclosed the sexual abuse at home, she was believed by her mental health clinicians, who called the child protection social workers to see and assess her. The two social workers who visited Mai assessed the situation and believed Mai's account of her father's behaviour. The child protection social workers found a foster placement for Mai, and the matter was referred to the police. Mai didn't want to live with a foster family, and, while her psychotic symptoms dissipated upon hospital discharge when she was transferred to live with a foster family, she became more depressed and withdrawn.

The mental health services then were in lockdown with the rest of the country, and so the social workers returned Mai to her family, as her father had moved out of the home. Despite follow-up counselling with the child protection social workers, Mai decided not to press charges and did not wish to appear in court to give evidence against her father. She retracted her disclosure in order to return her life to the status quo. Her father returned to the home soon after Mai retracted her statement. The charges were dropped, and her father moved back to the family home where they were once again in lockdown conditions together.

Table 7.1 summarises the risks and protective factors present in the case of Mai.

Reflections on the case study of Mai

The contents of the hallucinations were a form of disclosure before the words could be said or the letter written to her father telling him how she felt about his inappropriate touching. The period of being locked down with her family raised the terror of being victimised more frequently, so prompting a crisis for Mai. In hospital, she engaged with caring professionals who believed her story and acted upon it to establish her safety.

Despite the protective factor of having mental health professionals involved and believing her, the value of family in Middle Eastern culture was underestimated by the helping professionals involved. Mai was then in the position of

Table 7.1 Risk and protective factors in the case of Mai

Protective factors supporting disclosure as an adolescent/child	*Risk factors hampering disclosure as a child/adolescent*	*Life event(s) triggering initial disclosure*	*Outcome of disclosure*
Came to see the behaviour of her father as being 'sexual abuse'	Suicidal ideation Psychosis Self-harming behaviour (cutting arms to self soothe)	Psychosis and suicidality as unintentional way of telling others of her abuse Emergency department saw her and referred her for inpatient care	Retraction of disclosure Left foster placement
Realised her family patterns of communication and interaction were dysfunctional	Belief that father was head of the household and should be respected and honoured by all	Arabic culture has taboos on disclosing family matters to uphold the honour of the family	Returned to live with her family
Realised her mother would not listen to her	Father the financial breadwinner	The 'pressure cooker' effect led to unintentional disclosure	Family restored status quo
Health professionals directly asked and intervened	Economic dependence on father	Mai had been at risk during COVID-19 lockdown restrictions as it gave her father more opportunity to molest her	Mai in a situation of ongoing risk of abuse
Child protection intervened and foster care placement was organised	Mai anticipated that her mother would favour her father	Schools not open during COVID-19, which deflected attention to the home and staying with family	

disturbing the tranquillity of the family home and challenged the status of her father as head of the household. This brought much guilt to Mai and the abandonment by her mother. It was too difficult for her to uphold her disclosure as her mother pleaded for her forgiveness and minimised her abuse. The internal conflict led to her retraction of all allegations. Her position in her family as the eldest daughter meant that respect for her father and mother was non-negotiable. As studies of abuse disclosures in the Asian community have revealed, there are cultural mores surrounding fathers and the expectation that their offspring will demonstrate respect, whatever the father's behaviour towards them (Wahab et al., 2013). These traditional beliefs are also a feature of being a daughter in a Middle Eastern household (Timraz, et al., 2019). The lack of consistency in relationship to her caregivers when her three-week hospital stay ended had prompted a return to her predominant cultural worldview that meant she would be reunited with her family. Since she was again in a period of lockdown, she was likely to be at risk of retaliation from her father as well as her mother for her disclosure. Child protection social workers remained involved, though their involvement was limited by the COVID-19 restrictions to telephone contact.

Conclusion

Previous studies have found shame that survivors experience can be mediated through increased self-compassion, connection with others and disclosing and externalising shame and blame through learning about the abuse dynamics (Chouliara et al., 2014). Such studies recommend therapeutic interventions that work with the goal of mediating shame through externalising blame to avoid internalising shame. Removing self-blame is central to healing from historical sexual abuse. Shame can influence both the psychological and, ultimately, the physical dimensions of health, as the case studies of Makere and Jessie both illustrate. These findings portray the pervasive nature of shame following CSA as influencing survivors' adult lives across many domains of their life (MacGinley et al., 2019, p. 1143). Reductions in shame feature prominently in studies researching the lessening of PSTD symptoms in adult survivors of CSA. Such reductions were challenged by the restrictions on face-to-face interaction with those outside one's 'bubble' during the COVID-19 pandemic. These exclusions from contact therefore, included helping professionals. Further studies are needed to investigate the obstacles survivors feel to reaching out during global restrictions on contact with others during pandemics, such as those experienced during the COVID-19 lockdowns. Furthermore, for mind–body or holistic therapies to be available for women survivors and funded publicly necessitates a paradigm shift in the thinking that these domains are separate and discrete, when women survivors often see the division between mind and body as quite foreign. This becomes apparent when women survivors seek culturally specific, mind, body and spiritual therapies.

For women survivors who are First Nations people with experience of colonisation in their extended family narratives, culturally specific healing therapies may be required. Such therapies need to be publicly funded, and their availability should be more widely publicised. How the experience of cultural abuse, which may be intergenerational, interfaces with experiences of CSA needs to be further researched, as shame and discrimination can be interrelated and need gentle exploration with a culturally relevant therapist or healer.

The vicarious traumatisation of helping professionals can be more prominent when they are working remotely from a home-based practice as, without a support network of colleagues and the infrastructure of office equipment and resources, client issues and problems can seem all-encompassing (Buxton & Scudder, 2022). Working from home can bring these issues into the home, which can be seen as an infringement of the boundary between the personal and professional (Godlee, 2020).

In such circumstances, vicarious traumatisation can be a risk to the helping professionals working with CSA disclosures and material. Vicarious traumatisation is a term referring to the vicarious effects and impacts over time of engaging empathetically with sexual abuse trauma (Pearlman & Saakvitne, 1995). The potential for vicarious traumatisation is now recognised as being a normal part of the work with CSA survivors. Originally developed by the Traumatic Stress Institute in Connecticut, USA, the framework sees the self of the helper travelling a parallel path to that of the client(s) they are seeing for sexual abuse recovery work (Pearlman & Saakvitne, 1995).

In Chapter Eight, which concludes this book, we move on to explore more about vicarious traumatisation and how it can affect the practitioner's connection with the woman survivor of CSA. The chapter will discuss the implications for the practitioner's use of self in the therapeutic relationship with survivors of CSA. Professional self-care is a priority when therapists are themselves impacted by the grief of the global pandemic. Therefore, in the concluding chapter, recommendations for working with CSA disclosures at such times of heightened emotions are discussed, and recommendations are made. Similar conditions to those experienced during the COVID-19 pandemic are thought likely to recur in the future, and so it is not a matter of if, but rather when, these conditions are again encountered.

During the restrictions imposed by a global pandemic, connection may need to be made in a different way, so that the usual support options may be limited or non-existent. With the need to stay connected during such conditions to attend to what is happening with the client, the helping professional may be connected with clients virtually, at home. Thus, the concluding discussion, about the importance of maintaining professional boundaries and self-care as CSA disclosures are engaged with, is an important part of the ongoing need of clients to disclose what happened to them. This discussion will lead on to a summary of the themes of each chapter of the book as we turn to look at the key implications for practice with women survivors of CSA across the life course.

References

Alaggia, R., & Kirshenbaum, S. (2005). Speaking the unspeakable: exploring the impact of family dynamics on child sexual abuse disclosures. *Families in Society: The Journal of Contemporary Social Services*, 86(2), 227–234. doi:10.1606/1044-3894.2457

Azzopardi, C., Shih, C. S.-Y., Burke, A. M., Kirkland-Burke, M., Moddejonge, J. M., Smith, T. D., & Eliav, J. (2022). Supporting survivors of child sexual abuse during the COVID-19 pandemic: an ecosystems approach to mobilizing trauma-informed telemental healthcare. *Canadian Psychology/Psychologie canadienne*, 63(1), 43.

Butler, L. J., Lawton, A., & Kalali, P. (2023). Supporting survivors of institutional child sexual abuse during the COVID-19 pandemic: a qualitative study of not-for-profit community and legal organisations in Greater Western Sydney. *Australian Journal of Social Issues*, 58(4), 926–941.

Buxton, S., & Scudder, R. (2022). The importance of the supervisory relationship during adverse and unprecedented times. *Dramatherapy*, 43(1–3),16–32.

Chouliara, Z., Karatzias, T., & Gullone., A. (2014). Recovering from childhood sexual abuse: a theoretical framework for practice and research. *Mental Health Nursing*, 21(1), 69–78.

Gasker, J. A. (1999). *I Never Told Anyone This Before: Managing the Initial Disclosure of Sexual Abuse Re-Collections.* Psychology Press.

Gausman, J., & Langer, A. (2020). Sex and gender disparities in the COVID-19 pandemic. *Journal of Women's Health*, 29(4), 465–466.

Godlee, F. (2020). Trust is crucial in lockdown – and beyond. *BMJ*, 369. doi:10.1136/bmj.m1721

Kofman, Y. B., & Garfin, D. R. (2020). Home is not always a haven: the domestic violence crisis amid the COVID-19 pandemic. *Psychological Trauma: Theory, Research, Practice, and Policy*. doi:10.1037/tra0000866

MacGinley, M., Breckenridge, J., & Mowll, J. (2019). A scoping review of adult survivors' experiences of shame following sexual abuse in childhood. *Health Soc Care Community*, 27, 1135–1146. doi:10.1111/ hsc.12771

Mazza, M., Marano, G., Lai, C., Janiri, L., & Sani, G. (2020). Danger in danger: interpersonal violence during COVID-19 quarantine. *Psychiatry Research*, 289. doi:10.1016/j.psychres.2020.113046

McElvaney, R. (2015). Disclosure of child sexual abuse: delays, non-disclosure and partial disclosure. What the research tells us and implications for practice. *Child Abuse Review*, 24(3), 159–169. doi:10.1002/car.2280

McElvaney, R., Green, S., & Hogan, D. (2014). To tell or not to tell? Factors influencing young people's informal disclosures of child sexual abuse. *Journal of Interpersonal Violence*, 29(5), 928–947.

New Scientist. (2020). 11 July issue. No author.

Pearlman, L. A., & Saakvitne, K. W. (1995). *Trauma and the Therapist: Countertransference and Vicarious Traumatization in Psychotherapy with Incest Survivors*. W. W. Norton.

Roesch, E., Amin, A., Gupta, J., & García-Moreno, C. (2020). Violence against women during covid-19 pandemic restrictions. *BMJ*, 369. doi:10.1136/bmj.m1712

Timraz, S., Lewin, L., Giurgescu, C., & Kavanaugh, K. (2019). An exploration of coping with childhood sexual abuse in Arab American women. *Journal of Child Sexual Abuse*, 28(3), 360–381. doi:10.1080/10538712.2018.1538174

Tsur, N., & Abu-Raiya, H. (2020). COVID-19-related fear and stress among individuals who experienced child abuse: the mediating effect of complex posttraumatic stress disorder. *Child Abuse and Neglect*, 110(2). doi:10.1016/j.chiabu.2020.104694

Usher, K., Bhullar, N., Durkin, J., Gyamfi, N., & Jackson, D. (2020). Family violence and COVID-19: increased vulnerability and reduced options for support. *International Journal of Mental Health Nursing*. doi:10.1111/inm.12735

Van Berkel, S. R., Prevoo, M. J. L., Linting, M., Pannebakker, F. D., & Alink, L. R. A. (2020). Prevalence of child maltreatment in the Netherlands: an update and cross-time comparison. *Child Abuse and Neglect*, 103. doi:10.1016/j.chiabu.2020.104439

Van Gelder, N., Peterman, A., Potts, A., O'Donnell, M., Thompson, K., Shah, N., & Oertelt-Prigione, S. (2020). COVID-19: reducing the risk of infection might increase the risk of intimate partner violence. *EClinicalMedicine*, 21.

Wahab, S., Rahman, F. N. A., Mohd Hashim, S., & Razali, S. (2013). Intrafamilial sexual abuse in an Asian society: understanding the victim's internal conflicts. *International Medical Journal*, 20(2), 186–187. www.scopus.com/inward/record.uri?eid=2-s2.0-84878281572&partnerID=40&md5=ff493b0a2085e812e9070448bc0453dd

Wilson, D., Moloney, E., Parr, J. M., Aspinall, C., & Slark, J. (2021). Creating an Indigenous Māori-centred model of relational health: a literature review of Māori models of health. *Journal of Clinical Nursing*, 30(23–24), 3539–3555. doi:10.1111/jocn.15859

Wright, E. N., Miyamoto, S., & Richardson, C. (2022). The impact of COVID-19 restrictions on victim advocacy agency utilization across Pennsylvania. *Journal of Family Violence*, 37(6), 907–913. doi:10.1007/s10896-021-00307-z

8 Conclusion: a multidimensional approach to women's disclosure of CSA

Introduction

In this chapter, the themes of this book are drawn together to illuminate directions in practice with women survivors of CSA. This book began with the frameworks introduced in the first three chapters of trauma-informed, relational and attachment and narrative theory. In this chapter, we look at how these theories and directions in research have shaped our thinking about the disclosure of historical CSA by women survivors. To summarise the earlier literature reviews discussed throughout this book, there are five overarching themes identified for dealing with disclosure of historical CSA by women. These themes that have been identified are, first, an expanded definition of disclosure. The second theme is that of disclosure of CSA as an iterative process that occurs not as a single act of telling, but as a conversation over a lifetime. Third, disclosure is discussed as occurring in relation to a trusting relationship with another (or others). Fourth, the contextual factors that act singularly and together to facilitate or hinder disclosure are explored with reference to the risk and resilience literature. The risk and resilience literature explains why some children go on to thrive despite early traumatic experiences and childhood abuse, neglect and deprivation. Fifth, the limitations of previous research studies on disclosure of CSA will be overviewed. Lastly, the question of whether disclosure is necessary for recovery from CSA will be addressed on the basis of the literature reviewed.

The second part of this concluding chapter will draw together the principles of various theories presented throughout this book and apply these to what we have come to understand about disclosure, to form an integrated framework for practice with women survivors of CSA.

The theoretical approaches of New Trauma Therapy can be seen as laying the foundations for the current-day understanding of sexual abuse recovery and trauma-informed practice. Lessons from attachment and narrative theories will be identified; it will be argued that an understanding of aspects of each of these theories is needed for dealing with the disclosure of CSA. Finally the role of professional self-care and the potential for vicarious traumatisation (VT) will be raised, with suggestions for remaining open to fully

DOI: 10.4324/9781032669205-8

engaging with and actively listening to traumatic disclosures from women survivors who are presenting for help with their issues.

An expanded understanding of disclosure

Disclosure is the act of the woman survivor of CSA telling another, verbally or in writing, about her experiences of CSA in the past. Based on the literature and the case studies presented throughout this book, an expanded definition of disclosure is highlighted as being essential, as the telling of an abuse narrative to another involves an ongoing relationship in which to discuss the impact of the CSA on the woman survivor's life over her lifetime. Retrospective accounts of abuse given by adult women are usually delayed, with most historical disclosures of CSA being paused until the woman is over the age of 18 and with most disclosures happening when the woman is in her 20s or 30s (Mooney & McGregor, 2018). By this age, with increasing independence from one's family of origin where the abuse may have occurred or a negative response to a first telling may have been received, there are usually further opportunities to disclose in trusting adult relationships that have developed. A proportion of adult survivors will not disclose to anyone owing to cultural taboos and social mores, and the majority of disclosures are made informally to others rather than to child protection services or legal authorities in a search for active intervention or compensation (McElvaney, 2015).

Some theorists include behaviour or actions in the definition of disclosure of CSA, when verbal options are seen by the woman survivor either as not available and/or not possible owing to the level of distress she is experiencing (Alaggia, 2004). Alternatively, there can be a storing-up of emotions related to the abuse that precipitates a crisis in the present (McElvaney, 2015). 'Acting out' or behavioural manifestations are common in adolescence owing, in some instances, to immaturity and felt powerlessness to express what happened verbally. The case study of Mai was an illustration of what McElvaney (2015) has termed 'the pressure cooker effect'.

Disclosure as an iterative process

Rather than disclosure being a one-off event, current thinking has reconceptualised disclosure of CSA by women as involving a gradual recognition and acknowledgement (Alaggia, 2004). The decision to disclose then involves a choice point where a current life theme presents an opportunity to disclose for the first time or, alternatively, to disclose again. The decision making process to disclose or not is often based on a re-authoring process that the survivor engages in over time (White, 1995). I have conceptualised these moments, where a telling or a retelling is considered by survivor, as occurring in a 'liminal space', a term used in cultural anthropology and applied in narrative thinking about how trauma in the past is integrated into people's lives (Myerhoff, 1992). 'Liminal spaces' are pauses in the usual life narrative where the present life presents a need to integrate the past from which we learn, and a future can be imagined, but which may not yet be fully formed or realised. Within such spaces, the woman survivor is presented with an opportunity for telling and retelling her original abuse story. When memories from the past emerge and impact one's life in the present, this is another opportunity to retell the CSA narrative including the present alongside the past. In this process of telling or iteration, the survivor's knowledge and understanding of her abuse and its impact may grow, so expanding the survivor's awareness of what happened and its impact upon her life subsequently. Therefore, there can be a discursive process involved in repeated cycles of disclosure, with each disclosure changing what is known by the survivor about fragmented memories of CSA that may coalesce in the telling to another.

A relational approach to the disclosure of CSA

The story of abuse in childhood and its ongoing impact grows with the telling and retelling in relationship to a trusted other. When trust has been violated in the past, it can be a leap of faith for the survivor to trust another again. This is particularly so when a disclosure of CSA has been met by disbelief, scepticism or minimisation by significant others in the woman's childhood. Differing styles of attachment may be evident in the woman's early relationships with parents, family members and caregivers. These patterns of attachment can continue into adolescence and adulthood.

Disclosure assumes a relational quality that ideally facilitates ongoing support for the woman survivor throughout the process of retelling her story of CSA. Ideally, this relationship is forged and maintained through the formation and maintenance of a secure attachment that is experienced over time. Relationship and attachment are the mechanisms through which the survivor is supported towards embarking on disclosure of CSA as a reflective, iterative process as an adult. If the quality of the relationship is untrusting, blaming of the woman or inconsistent, opportunities for disclosure may not be recognised and engaged with. The challenge of each life stage often presents with a need to address one's narrative again, until patterns are discerned, and this knowledge becomes integrated into one's current life and identity.

Contextual factors supporting disclosure

As discussed in previous chapters, the conditions needed to safely disclose CSA depend on a constellation of factors that operate together, balancing various risks. These contextual factors often interrelate, and, when they come together as a whole, the protective factors can balance the cumulative risk factors. When these protective factors coalesce, the survivor may feel they have the background conditions to embark on a journey of retrospective disclosure of CSA.

Some of the major obstacles and barriers are summarised in Figure 8.1.

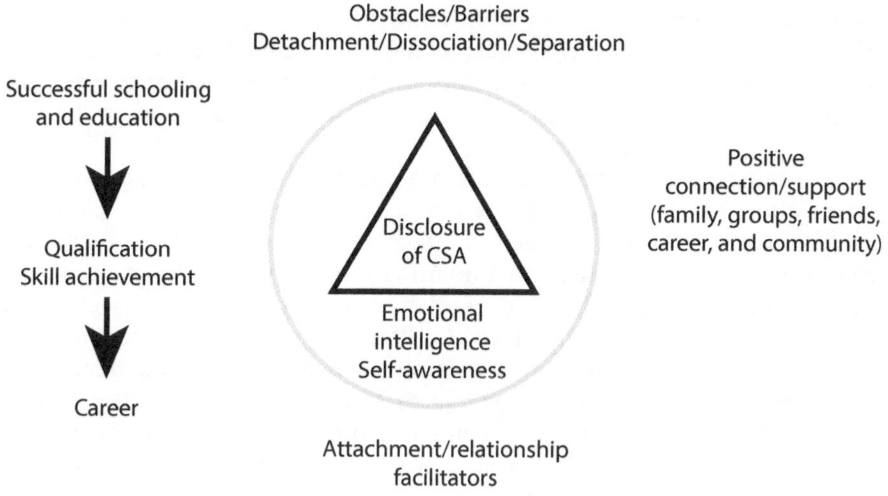

Figure 8.1 Factors influencing disclosure through the life span

These factors belong to three main categories that represent barriers or facilitators to disclosure as an adult. First, there are the factors relating to the individual resources of the woman; second, her social networks and their ability to provide connection and relationship; if they don't have this ability, isolation and disconnection may be features of her adult life; and third, the achievements and gains made in earlier life stages, resulting in a framework for quality of life throughout the rest of her adult years. To summarise:

1. Factors based on the individual: emotional intelligence, capacity to self-reflect, health, self-awareness, dissociation
2. Interpersonal factors: relationship, connection or separation leading to social isolation. Connection may be with professional others, such as counsellors, therapists or groups, or with friends, siblings, adult parents, peers, partners and adult children and in communities of interest and/or local community/culture
3. Life trajectory-related factors: achievement in earlier stages in terms of educational contexts, resulting in qualifications, career, housing and income. The time at which one was born and was growing up is significant in this dimension. The social mores and taboos about sexual abuse and the disclosure of CSA can feature as facilitators and/or obstacles in this dimension of life

Often, the support of a significant other (or others) and a secure attachment provide a safety net for disclosure to be made and the aftermath dealt with constructively, with the survivor controlling the pace and pathway for seeking help. For adolescents, recent research has discovered that behaviour and unintentional acting out can be a form of unconscious disclosure when the conditions are unfavourable to recognising abuse and feeling safe to disclose (Cossar et al., 2019). If teens had a trusting relationship with their professional significant other, who was often a youth worker or teacher, and this professional noticed something concerning in the young person's behaviour, this provided the 'good enough' mother (Winnicott, 1965) or caregiver relationship in which to disclose. Enquiring into the well-being of the young person in the context of this kind of relationship brought forth disclosure of current or earlier CSA (Cossar et al., 2019). When the authors asked, in interviews with a sample of young people, what precipitated intentional disclosure, it was often after the young person had assessed if it was safe to talk. The factors supporting conscious disclosure were the availability of a trusting relationship that the young person assessed over time as being 'safe', a positive response to disclosure and help seeking in the past, and recognition of the perpetrator's behaviour being sexual abuse. A particular worry for the teens interviewed was splitting the family up through their disclosure, meaning that, when the perpetrator was a family member, the abuse was more likely to remain hidden or the telling would be significantly delayed (Cossar et al., 2019).

Findings from the risk and resilience literature

Resilience literature is predicated on the idea that, in formative years, an individual develops internal psychological resources to meet fundamental needs and to cope with the demands of later life. One of the challenges to developmental psychology is to explain why some children are at risk, and why the buffering conditions protect some children but not others, despite helpful family and home environments (Luthar, 1991).

A further area in which the risk and resilience literature is informative about the factors influencing disclosure is when cumulative protective factors are present. Protective factors have been discovered to act similarly to cumulative risks – that is, in developing what has been referred to as 'cumulative protection' (Fraser et al., 1999). The notion that cumulative protection enables individuals to develop adaptive responses buffering negative ones has a more optimistic orientation. For example, some, studies suggest that vulnerability factors are not long-standing experiences but are, rather, key moments relating to choice points in peoples' lives (Rutter, 1987). Second, cumulative protection has been associated with the development of alternative belief systems and personal philosophies. These personal philosophies are thought to develop with experience and are learned abilities that develop over time (Fraser et al., 1999).

Those writing from relational perspectives have challenged the idea that resilience exists for reasons of individual personality or the social resources surrounding the individual. Resilience is thought to be grounded in a two-way process of giving and receiving that has its origins in the establishment of trust in another and the quality of the individual survivor's relationships with others. Consequently, resilience can involve a community, whether this be online in the #MeToo sense or a support network of peers, colleagues, friends and supporters.

Obstacles to disclosure – culture, social stigma and the potential for internalised shame

The factors that impede, slow or derail the disclosure of CSA have been summarised as involving the woman's experience of past attempts at disclosure of CSA and how these disclosures were met by the person disclosed to. Age-related, cultural and social taboos about disclosing childhood sexual abuse are prominent in the literature about the obstacles to disclosure. It is thought that these negative factors are often internalised by the woman herself, so preventing any attempt at disclosure of CSA at all, as we saw illustrated in the case study of Alice. Delayed disclosure may be left to adulthood and, in some cases, close to the end of the woman's life owing to these factors involving societal and familial attitudes.

Culture and social stigma

The variables of culture and the predominant cultural and historical beliefs of the time in which the survivor was raised may determine whether disclosure is even considered as an option by the woman survivor. Given these relational and socio-cultural complexities surrounding the decision of the survivor to disclose or not, the issue of whether disclosure is necessary from the perspective of the woman survivor of CSA is raised. In the previous research reviewed in this book, at the time of writing, this question had yet to be fully answered. This is owing to the multifactorial considerations and life trajectories detailed throughout this book and illustrated in the case studies. Historical disclosure by adult survivors may not be made owing to the complexity of the disclosure process itself. Second, some supportive factors may be present and others not, and the interaction of these factors when taken together form a constellation that supports disclosure or not. Therefore, it is difficult to look at such factors individually, as they usually do not exist in isolation as favoured in experimental research designs. Third, despite overwhelming obstacles, some adult survivors go on to thrive when disclosure may not have been made. This follows the risk and resiliency literature showing that not all life trajectories are derailed by early trauma such as CSA and a lack of disclosure.

Unlike for other traumas, social stigma is still attached to survivors telling of their abuse narrative and how it has influenced their lives. The degree of stigma can be socially and culturally bound and, when it operates, can have the effect of militating against disclosure, often over the woman's entire lifespan. The act of telling is potentially risky, as in the scenario where the survivor is disbelieved or ridiculed for what she has told the other. This negative feedback can begin a self-blaming cycle where shame and negative self-talk dominate a woman's life, promoting less positive outcomes. For example entering adult relationships that mirror the original abuse dynamics by involving psychological or physical harm to the survivor, have been previously documented. Disruptions of education, impacting career and income earning potential, have been found in prior research involving women survivors of CSA. The extended case narrative of Shelia and her partner Rob looked at the legacy of sexual abuse across a lifespan where there was a balancing of risk and resiliency factors operating. The influence of the ongoing impact of CSA on women's decision making about fertility, pregnancy and parenting is evident in the case studies across women's reproductive lifespan, as illustrated in the case studies of the women survivors in Chapters Two, Three and Four.

In summary, whether disclosure is therapeutic in its after-effects from women survivors' perspectives depends on a host of factors. The first group of these factors, as identified by Ullman et al. (2010), concerns how far disclosure is shared with others or kept to the survivor herself; the nature of the response to disclosure; and the nature of the disclosure itself in terms of how it is told (in writing or verbally) and whether recounted as fact and in terms of the intensity of the emotional content of the telling. The characteristics of the discloser, how far disclosure is voluntary or offered, the relationship to those disclosed to, the length of time since the sexual abuse, and the gender of the person disclosed to and their current psychological functioning are other documented variables (Ullman et al., 2010, p. 150).

Cossar et al. (2019) concur with these differing trajectories and identify, in their research, several categories of disclosure. They categorise telling oneself only as disclosure that remains hidden and disclosure as an act where the survivor engages with various kinds of risk taking behaviour (i.e., manifested in different forms of signs and symptoms). They categorise 'prompted telling' where a supportive other listens attentively and may make a general observation that there is a change they have noticed in the survivor. Lastly, they categorise 'purposeful telling' where the survivor actively seeks out a helping professional to deal with the aftermath of CSA.

The overarching socio-cultural factors are variables influencing whether disclosure is helpful or likely to isolate, or bring shame or attract retribution to the survivor for the telling. Shame attributed to the woman survivor in some cultures can be so negative that women survivors may become acutely unwell in the distress of having to keep their abuse hidden and, when the opportunity to disclose comes, it poses a dilemma. The case study of Mai illustrated these factors from within a Middle Eastern Arabic perspective. Acknowledging the CSA by talking about it to others can precipitate a life crisis the effects of which can be wide-ranging. The mental health issues can range from psychosis to depression (Wahab et al., 2013).

In the case study of Stella, who was from a Pasifika cultural background, her disclosure to her aunt was a strong protective factor in her sexual abuse trauma, after she had been disbelieved by her mother. The extent of her abuse at the hands of her stepfather and its nature meant that she had developed ways of coping through detaching herself from her body. Dissociation is discussed as a common coping strategy, conceptualised by the New Trauma therapists as being both contextual to childhood sexual abuse and mediated by the woman survivor's existing repertoire of coping mechanisms to deal day-to-day with the re-experiencing of sexual abuse trauma as an adult (Briere, 1996; Courtois, 1997; Dalenberg, 2000; Herman, 1992). The therapist's or helping professional's understanding of the existence of protective factors and of how they can operate to balance risk factors in the woman survivor's life at any one time is imperative for understanding her journey of healing from CSA. Second, attending to her developed adaptations and coping strategies for dealing with past CSA to find ways of honouring what the woman has developed in her life is an underlying theme of trauma-informed theory with its origins in the theory of sexual abuse recovery (Briere, 1996; Courtois, 1997; Dalenberg, 2000; Herman, 1992).

Limitations of previous research into disclosure

More recent research into disclosure of CSA has found some deficits in the methodology of previous studies. Past research into disclosure of CSA has tended to use experimental designs with controlled populations of participants being interviewed, surveyed or observed in a controlled setting, such as a clinic or with captive audiences (Ullman et al., 2010). Many research studies employed university students as participants, as much academic research happens in a university context and students are an available population and willing to be researched.

The prevailing research design of these studies and the over-representation of students within these studies have meant the many social and environmental factors that inevitably impact upon disclosure of CSA have remained hidden and unaddressed (Ullman et al., 2010). These contextual factors have been researched more widely in recent years and written about as background factors that have the effect of either hindering or facilitating disclosure. These 'moderators and mediators' of disclosure (Ullman et al., 2010) form an evidence base from which practitioners working in the field of sexual abuse recovery can usefully draw. This evidence base of the contextual factors conducive to safe disclosure by women survivors sits within the broader risk and resiliency literature reviewed in Chapter One. This risk and resiliency literature explains why some individuals are able to survive and go on to thrive as adults despite early histories of childhood adversity and trauma. Hitherto, it was assumed that the impact of childhood trauma would be universally negative and influence poor outcomes in adult life to a larger extent. This literature is connected to the contextual factors supporting disclosure, as the wider risk and resilience literature emphasises the importance of a significant relationship in the child's life. It is the supportive relationship that serves as a protective factor in the presence of multiple risks, including sexual abuse and maternal neglect or lack of safe attachment. Such a relationship can also be a buffer to the attitude of disbelief about the abuse from the non-offending parent/guardian.

Is disclosure supportive of women's healing from CSA?

Underlying many of the practice-based studies is an assumption that there are positive benefits to the survivor of disclosing historical CSA. A qualifier to this discussion is that disclosure is perhaps only constructive from the survivor's perspective when the wider family and life stage conditions support the ongoing process of disclosure. Outcome studies involving adult women's disclosure of CSA affirm the positive legacy of disclosure, beginning with the 'talking therapy' established by Freudian psychoanalysis (Freud, 1909). Although Freud later repudiated the veracity of women's disclosure of incest during the process of 'free association', this denial of the harsh realities of his women patients' lives is now thought to be due to the social mores of his day. The underlying object relations approach to engaging women survivors in disclosure was established, nonetheless, and the theoretical grounding for psychodynamic therapies developed through the process of Freud's 'free association'. Within psychodynamic approaches, there are styles of relating established, knowledge of which can be useful for women's healing from CSA.

Relational psychotherapies based on attachment theory are predicated on the understanding that the women's positive experience of disclosing recollections of CSA occurs when the disclosures are witnessed by a supportive, non-judgemental professional other. The process of being affirmed in the presence of another creates a relationship within which further reflection about the impact of CSA on one's life can, subsequently, be made safely. Through a secure attachment bond, the therapeutic relationship is thought to create a buffer, built by the therapeutic rapport, to mitigate various risk factors such as the survivor's internalising stress and trauma or becoming re-traumatised through recalling the original experience of CSA. The therapeutic relationship can become a strong protective factor in disclosure, therefore, even in the face of previous negative responses to disclosure from others. Key variables are readiness to engage in the therapeutic relationship and the professional's expertise in forming and sustaining an ongoing rapport with the adult woman survivor of CSA.

Ullman et al. (2010) reviewed earlier studies that have linked the wider health benefits of disclosure of past trauma positively affecting the immune system and physical well-being. Disclosure in the context of a trusting therapeutic relationship is thought to promote less negatively impacted and more productive lives for women survivors in a psychological sense. This positive spiral is thought to be accomplished through the act of disclosure, whether this be to significant others, family or helping professionals (Ullman et al., 2010).

From the New Trauma therapists to trauma-informed theory

As previously discussed, this engagement with disclosure of CSA often involves past iterations of the client's life narrative as well as the current presenting issue triggering a telling or retelling of the actual events or the ongoing grief at the effects of CSA. This book has proposed the usefulness of a narrative systems framework through which practitioners and supporters of women survivors can better understand the multidimensional nature of CSA's effects across the life lived.

Second, a relational perspective needs to be included in the helping professional's repertoire of theories for working with women CSA survivors. For example, the lessons learned through working within the restrictions to face-to-face contact during the global COVID-19 pandemic have intensified the search for appropriate platforms that offer opportunities for therapeutic attachment. Without a safe attachment to another, facilitating disclosure of CSA for the therapist and the client, who may both be at home with their families and significant others when this work is underway, is in question. How, then, professionals effectively connect with their client's efforts at disclosure assumes a therapeutic relationship that offers a 'good enough' relationship (Winnicott, 1965). This relational focus of New Trauma Therapy incorporates a social justice perspective promoting advocacy and information sharing in the therapeutic work.

A narrative approach is important during life transitions when there is a movement from the familiar and the known and survivors find they are facing new challenges and milestones. The woman survivor who is facing such challenges can be catapulted into 'liminal spaces' of betwixt and between where the known is no longer relevant and the development of new directions requires a re-authoring process (White, 1995).

In summary, an eclectic mix of theoretical approaches is needed to see the therapeutic task more broadly. This theoretical diversity, together with ongoing exposure to traumatic material, can mean that helping professionals engaging with trauma can themselves become desensitised over time. Therefore, an understanding of vicarious traumatisation and professional self-care is needed in the engagement with women survivors of CSA (Pack, 2016).

A multi-theoretical approach to disclosure

The approaches to working with women survivors around the issues of disclosure are both multi-theoretical and multidimensional. An early assessment of past responses to disclosure to family/significant others is essential to understanding delays in seeking help for CSA issues.

There should be an assessment of the balance of risk and protective factors operating in the survivor's life, including an understanding of the phase of life the survivor is in and the current challenges of this phase. The responses to attempts to disclose also need to be assessed. Lastly, the ability of the helping professional to be present emotionally to engage and listen fully to what the woman is saying is central to CSA recovery work. Such a relationship provides a safe container for witnessing disclosure, which attachment theorists and trauma-informed theory deem to be critical to disclosure and to the healing process. Overall, for retrospective disclosure of CSA to be engaged in by women survivors, there will be an assessment as to whether the risks outweigh the protective factors in retelling their CSA story to another. If the risks are more prominent, then the survivor will tend not to disclose for the first time or choose to disclose again (Alaggia, 2004; Alaggia, 2005).

Theoretical approaches that attend to context and encompass principles of social justice

As described in Chapter One, the trauma-informed theory we know today began to be established by the founding theorists of New Trauma Therapy of the late 1980s and 1990s. Earlier on, a feminist self-help orientation arising from social ferment after the Vietnam War and the influence of the feminist movement brought the needs of survivors of all forms of traumatic experience to the general public's attention. War veterans returning from the Vietnam War focused more attention on the need for survivors of trauma to have access to opportunities for disclosure of the effects of the war on them and to revisit past trauma over time, as the impact became apparent. Here, the concept of 'bearing with' the client's ongoing need for trauma disclosure in an iterative way is suggested (Herman, 1992).

Themes from the psychobiology of trauma suggest that there are biological foundations for the helping professional's need to 'bear with' and to 'bear witness to' trauma in the adult survivor's recovery from traumatic events (Herman, 1992; Briere, 1996). These theorists and later researchers have found that human beings process traumatic material in a different way and in a different area of the brain from non-traumatic material. Telling one's CSA story enables the brain to integrate the raw, emotional memory into a history or narrative, known as the development of 'biographical memory' (Herman, 1992) to make sense of the material. If therapists are dealing with fragments of traumatic memory – both material triggered by their own experiences and material brought into the therapy room by clients – there needs to be a parallel processing of memory from the emotional or primitive part of the brain to the part of the brain that integrates the material into a history or narrative (Herman, 1992). Talking about a traumatic experience enables the client and the therapist to develop an ability to integrate the material encountered in the context of the therapeutic relationship. If there is not a way of moving from the traumatic, fragmented memory to cognitive memory, the client and the therapist are unlikely to be able to integrate the material disclosed in therapy or to take positive steps forward. Progress in therapy may be impeded if both the therapist and client are engaged in a parallel process of being immobilised by traumatic material or if there is insufficient emotional engagement by the therapist (Wilson & Lindy, 1994). The development of the psychobiological literature has had the effect of removing the stigma from trauma by focusing on the underlying processes involved and the positive life outcomes possible. For example, schooling from childhood through to higher degree learning is discussed as being a protective factor for women's CSA. The establishment of this educational trajectory can lead to further educational achievements, academic qualifications and well-paid work. Having enough money to meet one's expenses, which is often linked to educational attainment and career, was discussed in the research studies as being a strongly protective factor buffering more negative ones such as a history of CSA in one's family.

Attachment as the process underlying the survivors' relationships

One of the protective factors most often cited in the risk and resilience literature as a facilitator of disclosure is the availability of a relationship with a trusted other providing a 'secure base' of ongoing support. A professional who is assisting the woman in her healing joins this community of engaged others or may be the only person who has been witness to this disclosure. In the case study of Shelia in Chapter Five on midlife, we explored the case study of an adult survivor of CSA who had a life narrative that revolved around her relationship with her partner Rob, from high school until the present day. Although she lacked a secure base at home, school and her peer relationships (two associated protective factors) worked to buffer the more detrimental effects of CSA in her child hood and as an adolescent in institutional care. Her truancy was a form of unintentional disclosure that something was 'wrong' at home, and this was picked up by the school and brought to the attention of the authorities. She chose not to tell about feeling uncomfortable at home and the reasons for this, but her peers and teachers were aware and listened to her distress. Her subsequent abuse in foster care was discussed with a girlfriend and her family, who brought the issues to the authorities. The importance and role of peer relationships are an under-researched area and are worthy of further investigation.

Life stage triggering a need for disclosure and re-disclosure across the life course

The life phase itself can trigger the need to tell or tell another again about one's recollections of CSA. These times include some events that are age- and stage-specific. These ages and stages are not meant to be prescriptive but are representative of opportunities for exploring the impact of CSA in one's life again.

In Chapter One, the case study of Fiona and her wish for financial compensation for her experience of CSA was the first case of historical CSA I had encountered in my career, which began as a mental health professional. When I met her, Fiona was in the middle of a personal crisis that arose in the context of her life goals (home ownership and financial independence) when she was having difficulty managing anxiety as a young adult which was affecting her job security. Her primary presentation was framed as needing to manage her anxiety day-to-day as she was referred to the community mental health services.

Looking back now, this referral to the mental health services was potentially pathologising, as complex PTSD is a commonly experienced response to a history of child sexual abuse. The silence about her abuse up to this point highlighted the significance of societal attitudes about the family and what happens within it as being an essentially private space. Prevailing societal attitudes, reinforced by the silence of the survivor who assesses it is unsafe to tell, underline the fact that what happens in one's childhood owing to internal family norms generally is not intended to be discussed in the public gaze or to attract public intervention. As Fiona had requested a report to accompany her claim for compensation, some personal details of her abuse and its impact were inevitably needed subsequently to substantiate her eligibility for public funding of compensation for her CSA. During her disclosure of some of the details needed for her claim for compensation, her CSA triggered a remembering of abuse by the perpetrator. In the relative safety of the relationship with me, Fiona remembered and, in this process, projected details associated with her stepmother on to me, as the witness to her abuse narrative.

In Chapter Two, the life course model was introduced within a narrative framework. Decisions about having children represent a potential trigger for CSA tellings and retellings to arise. Pregnancy, with the bodily changes occurring, can signal women's need to discuss CSA issues. Anxiety about protecting one's child from CSA to avoid a pattern of intergenerational abuse means that the pressure is on to be the parent that the survivor lacked in her own life. The case study of Lisa and her longing to be the mother she never had throughout her life raised again memories of CSA. The birth experience can also evoke memories of the abuse, and birth planning is advised with a personalised approach and relationship with treating doctors and midwives. Where pregnancy loss brings an acute grief response, the grieving can include the lack of mothering and protection in the CSA experience. The notion of an epiphany or a breakthrough in making connections between the present loss and the past CSA can integrate the past trauma within the present crisis.

In Chapter Three, we discussed how the later adolescent period of forging first romantic relationships can bring challenges to the fore that hitherto remained hidden. Young women survivors of CSA have been found to have a sense, in their earlier life, of their abuse, with a generalised sense of something being wrong. They may not see the full import of what has happened to them as being sexual abuse. Alternatively, cultural taboos can mean that abuse remains hidden and undisclosed to anyone but the survivor herself. Disclosure may come about because a significant other has listened or reflected to them that there has been a change in their behaviour that is of concern to them. Acting out, such as self-harm or suicidality, is one way in which help is being sought without conscious acts of disclosure. The case study of Stella illustrates many of these dilemmas when she found a partner and was trying to forge a longer-term relationship with him.

In Chapter Four, the impact of the break-up of a relationship on a survivor of CSA (Kayla), who became acutely suicidal and self-harming, was explored. She felt pessimistic about ever finding the love she had longed for throughout her life after an infidelity and a betrayal of her on social media. Her distress was impacting her self-esteem and employment as she was thinking of leaving her job. Kayla moved from an independent living situation to return to live with her parents, which seemed like a backward step to her, and she became hopeless about her future. During her supportive counselling, she came to retell her abuse story in the context of reviewing all of her past romantic relationships and, in this retelling, found some solace. It prompted a disclosure to her ex-partner's mother of her son's behaviour. A relationship of trust grew between her and her mother-in-law, who supported Kayla's recovery subsequently. This compassionate response and relationship with her mother-in-law assisted Kayla towards feeling she had a future with another relationship.

In Chapter Four, we also saw decision making around parenting in the case study of Roz. The decision to try for a pregnancy in the hope of having children is prominent for women throughout the reproductive lifespan. For women today, the decision to delay parenting is part of the wider discussion about how to balance parenting with other roles, such as having a professional career. Dealing with a change of lifestyle from professional to full-time parent can be a difficult one, as being at home full time can be a normal transition but, for some survivors of CSA, the lack of control can prompt a life crisis as the adult woman survivor of CSA feels under pressure to be the parent she felt she had never had nor experienced herself as she was growing up.

The care from the professionals involved in an adult survivor's first pregnancy can be another time of transition when the need for disclosure of her history of CSA can become prominent. Sensitivity and a paced and collaborative approach to the care surrounding the woman survivor were needed. Giving the survivor an active role in developing a birth plan in conjunction with her midwife, nurses and doctors assisted the survivor with feeling more in control at a time when she was feeling very out of control. Following the birth, there were again periodic worries about mothering, but, with reassurance from midwives and further counselling, she was able to settle into the role.

In midlife, the focus can be on changes in career, primary relationships and parenting, as children grow and leave the family home, refocusing attention on a couple's relationship and future life goals, which might include planning towards retirement and a search for a better quality of life. The case study of Shelia in Chapter Five illustrates this time of transition, involving changing roles with the emptying of the nest when children left for university and facing her partner's health crisis. Couple work revealed that the worries that were arising for Shelia related to her being alone. This couple therapy led to a retelling of her abuse narrative in terms of how those experiences had affected their marriage. Through the partner being coached as witness to the retelling, their sense of their history together in the aftermath of the abuse was able to be explored. Furthermore, her partner was able to understand why she acted in certain ways towards him, which increased his understanding of the legacy of her abuse in the present. Together, they were able to grieve the losses to their intimacy based on the way Shelia had adapted to her abuse in adulthood.

In older age, matured insights about one's earlier life can influence a retelling of one's narrative, including the abuse narrative and how it impacted one's life across time. Chapter Six discussed the extended case study of Alice, who called me on a helpline for sexual abuse survivors; like many women survivors of her generation, she had chosen not to tell anyone of her abuse across her entire life. She did not wish for compensation, or to tell anyone else about her CSA, but this anonymous voice across a freephone provided safety to discuss what had happened to her. She did want, before the end of her life, to tell her family what had happened in terms of her long history of sexual abuse within her family of origin, as she had come to realise in her later years how her life had been impacted by her abuse. She wanted to explain to her sons and ex-husband why she was the way she was throughout their life together, and it was something that brought a sense of resolution to her present life.

The impact of COVID-19 restrictions on the retrospective disclosure of CSA

In Chapter Seven, the impact of the global pandemic was explored with the implications for supporting victims. During a time of national sorrow over the deaths of loved ones through COVID-19-related complications, this was a challenging time for women who were living in situations of isolation during government-mandated lockdowns that imposed restrictions on movement and contact with others, especially prior to the advent of vaccination against the different variations of the virus, which had unknown origins. This was a time of heightened anxiety about how to stay well and preserve one's well-being for the general populace. For survivors, there were often difficulties maintaining connection with helping professionals through remote platforms, as illustrated in the case studies of Jessie and Makere. In both case studies, there were difficulties obtaining health services linked to the health legacy of CSA. The two women were at different points in their life trajectory, with Jessie being in her 20s and Makere in her late 40s. Both women were challenged by their ineligibility for publicly funded services as adult survivors of CSA, and this triggered a crisis that mirrored not being believed about their original abuse and their need for health-related care to assist their recovery. The retelling of their abuse stories to media was an attempt to highlight difficulties in obtaining the care they needed.

As they both struggled with the remote technologies necessary during COVID-19 lockdown conditions, communication with their counsellor, case manager and other health professionals through remote and virtual platforms was inconsistent and introduced new obstacles to disclosing why they needed the services they were applying for. The need to deal with the whole person in terms of the physical, psychological and spiritual dimensions of care is not always recognised in health models that privilege the physical over the other dimensions of well-being. This narrow focus on the physical dimensions of health has been criticised by indigenous models of health care more recently, where responsibilities to respect the cultural diversity of women survivors have been emphasised, as cultural beliefs may make historical disclosure more difficult (Glover et al., 2010).

In New Zealand, responsibilities under the Treaty of Waitangi have meant that indigenous models are increasingly integrated into the health care services (Glover et al., 2010; Wilson et al., 2021) but may have been impeded by the difficulties of lack of face-to-face contact during COVID-19 restrictions. With the unknown impact of COVID-19, teams, individual practitioners, organisations and their surrounding institutions were challenged to provide new ways of connecting with women survivors of CSA, and the ability to remain relational was tested owing to the need to engage and work remotely, often from home. Organisations may have lacked access to remote technologies, and funding is needed to build infrastructure, as was the experience with the Sydney-based sexual abuse services in Australia during the COVID-19 pandemic (Butler et al., 2023).

The potential for VT and traumatic transference was found to be an everyday experience during the weeks and months of the pandemic, yet the supervisory relationship, which needed to remain clinically effective, faced similar challenges of remote technologies and working from home (Buxton & Scudder, 2022).

The case study of Mai illustrates that, sometimes, disclosure that does not go at the pace or in the direction the woman survivor wishes can re-traumatise, exacerbating the initial presentation. There were also the complication of lockdown and the difficulties of having to report historical CSA to the child protection authorities, when the adolescent was still living within the family in which they were abused. The survivor may not wish for disconnection from schooling or dislocation from her family with a move into statutory care. To be returned to her family of origin, Mai rescinded her original disclosure of CSA made to mental health professionals during an apparent psychotic episode.

Witnessing disclosure and vicarious traumatisation

As the relationship provides the crucible for healing from CSA, the self of the helping professional needs to be available to fully listen to the survivor. As discussed in previous chapters, VT features routinely in practitioners' engagement with traumatic disclosures. It relates to the changes in the experience of helping professionals as a consequence of their engagement with traumatic material that is disclosed in the therapeutic context (Pearlman & Saakvitne, 1995). Underpinned by constructivist self-development theory, the researchers of the Traumatic Stress Institute of Connecticut, USA, discovered that working with potentially traumatic material can have a range of identifiable impacts on the therapist in terms of worldview, belief systems, self-esteem and relationships. The cognitive constructs or thinking patterns and belief systems of therapists are thought to be permanently transformed by the cumulative impact of the work (McCann & Pearlman, 1990). Some of these cognitive transformations happen in an insidious way, so that the therapist may be unaware of the changes as they develop gradually over time. These changes can transform the therapist's personal relationships, sense of self and intimacy within close relationships. Isolation and withdrawal are common responses to the experience of VT, while connection, sense of community and absorbing interests and relationships ameliorate it.

In my research with sexual abuse therapists, this experience of VT was described to me as 'a baptism by fire' and was particularly noticed in the first five years of practice (Pack, 2004). The work and organisational environment were found to be central to therapists' sense of what was vicariously traumatising. The counsellors noticed, in the employing organisation's reporting requirements, a lack of attention to the context in which the abuse occurred. The public insurance scheme (ACC) they worked as contractors for asked them to work with individual claimants with focused goals, when the issues were very often long term and involved constructing a safe relationship in which to work therapeutically. Therefore, the dissonance of being asked to work in a cognitive behavioural way when the issues were relational, multigenerational and systemic in origin did not fit the way the therapists interviewed actually operated.

For the therapists who worked with woman survivors of CSA, there was an awareness of the issues surrounding the abuse inhering in the wider discourses of family, local community, culture and society. This need to see CSA as contextually and systemically based contrasted with the need to analyse and diagnose their clients who were women CSA survivors.

Disclosure of CSA is only a healing event if there is a supportive other to witness and fully hear the life narrative of the woman survivor and how her childhood abuse has impacted her life. If the therapist cannot engage empathetically with the woman and what she says, the conditions for disclosure and working with disclosure range from being ineffectual to being re-traumatising. Therefore, listeners need to be aware of the impacts of the nature of the work with sexual abuse disclosures on themselves and find ways of transforming these impacts creatively over their careers.

Clinical supervision, ongoing professional development/education and balancing the workload–caseload mix, where traumatic disclosures are tempered with more general referrals, have all been discovered to be helpful in ameliorating VT (Pack, 2016). With reference to the supervisory relationship, relational models of clinical supervision that allow free discussion on how the work is impacting one's life personally as well as professionally are important. I have conceptualised this quality of relationship as involving the personal and the professional, including an ongoing assessment of how the clinical work is impacting in relation to vicarious traumatisation and traumatic transference. Lastly, organisations that are hierarchical in structure and prescriptive in policy and protocols often do not allow therapists and other helping professionals to forge a therapeutic relationship sufficiently to allow for an exploration of CSA issues for women (Pack, 2004).

Conclusion and the way forward

The disclosure of CSA by women is central to our understanding of the prevalence of sexual abuse across cultures and across the life course. The research on disclosure explains why CSA is more extensive than we know about owing to the under-reporting of CSA in adulthood. The barriers of socio-cultural factors, family attitudes and upbringing, previous negative responses to disclosure prompting internalised shame and, lastly, systemic organisational, service and institutional failures have all been highlighted (Mooney & McGregor, 2018). Owing to these systemic, institutional and socio-cultural barriers, the disclosure of CSA is most often made less formally to health professionals, counsellors, psychotherapists, psychologists and social workers than to the legal fraternity, police and public inquiries. Owing to the many obstacles to talking about the abuse and its aftermath retrospectively as an adult, significant others who have a trusting, ongoing relationship with the survivor may be chosen as the safe haven in which to disclose historical abuse (Mooney & McGregor, 2018).

The process of disclosure is closely associated with understanding the ongoing nature of CSA and how CSA impacts survivors' lives over their lifetime. The life course perspective offers a means of understanding the complex, manifold nature of disclosure across life. The lived experiences of adult women and the role of disclosure of historical CSA over their lives are areas for future research.

One possible way through the barriers relating to systemic and service failure is finding a better system for women who, when making disclosures, have to tell their abuse story to several different agencies. While disclosure is largely seen as a therapeutic process in New Zealand, and a public insurance scheme (ACC) makes referrals to a counsellor, psychotherapist or psychologist to assess eligibility for a claim, perhaps this scope needs to be widened to allow the sharing (with client consent) of the claim-related information with the police and access to legal services if the woman wishes to seek redress for her CSA through the legal processes and courts.

Second, addressing the potential for the vicarious traumatisation of frontline helping professionals so that they stay present and engaged while witnessing disclosures from women survivors of CSA is imperative. If there is no one to hear fully what the woman survivor is disclosing, the potential for re-traumatising is heightened, particularly for women who received a negative response to their initial attempts to tell a significant other at earlier life stages. Lastly, the remote delivery of services to women survivors of CSA requires a technology infrastructure that facilitates, supports and guides women in complex systems in situations such as a global pandemic. There needs to be enough training on a range of theoretical models of practice so that practitioners feel informed, professionally and personally supported, and empathetic towards their clients. The stories of CSA may be hard to hear, but it is crucial that, as professionals, we are well prepared and proactively listening.

References

Alaggia, R. (2004). Many ways of telling: expanding conceptualizations of child sexual abuse disclosure. *Child Abuse and Neglect*, 28, 1213–1227.

Alaggia, R. (2005). Disclosing the trauma of child sexual abuse: a gender analysis. *Journal of Trauma and Loss*, 10(5), 453–470.

Briere, J. (1996). *Therapy for Adults Molested as Children: Beyond Survival*. Springer.

Butler, L. J., Lawton, A., & Kalali, P. (2023). Supporting survivors of institutional child sexual abuse during the COVID-19 pandemic: a qualitative study of not-for-profit community and legal organisations in Greater Western Sydney. *Australian Journal of Social Issues*, 58(4), 926–941.

Buxton, S., & Scudder, R. (2022). The importance of the supervisory relationship during adverse and unprecedented times. *Dramatherapy*, 43(1–3),16–32.

Cossar, J., Belderson, P., & Brandon, M. (2019). Recognition, telling and getting help with abuse and neglect: young people's perspectives. *Children and Youth Services Review*, 106. doi:10.1016/j.childyouth.2019.104469

Courtois, C. A. (1997). Healing the incest wound: a treatment update with attention to recovered-memory issues. *American Journal of Psychotherapy*, 51(4), 464–496. doi:10.1176/appi.psychotherapy.1997.51.4.464

Dalenberg, C. J. (2000). *Countertransference and the Treatment of Trauma*. American Psychological Association.

Fraser, M., Richman, J., & Galinsky, M. (1999). Risk, protection and resilience: toward a conceptual framework for social work practice . *Social Research*, 23, 131–143.

Freud, S. (1909). Five lectures on psycho-analysis. *SE*, 11.

Glover, D. A., Loeb, T. B., Carmona, J. V., Sciolla, A., Zhang, M., Myers, H. F., & Wyatt, G. E. (2010). Childhood sexual abuse severity and disclosure predict post-traumatic stress symptoms and biomarkers in ethnic minority women. *Journal of Trauma & Dissociation*, 11(2), 152–173.

Herman, J. L. (1992). *Trauma and Recovery*. New York: Basic Books.

Luthar, S. (1991). Vulnerability and resilience: a study of high risk adolescents. *Child Development*, 62, 600–616.

McCann, I. L., & Pearlman, L. A. (1990). Vicarious traumatization: a framework for understanding the psychological effects of working with victims. *Journal of Traumatic Stress*, 3, 131–149.

McElvaney, R. (2015). Disclosure of child sexual abuse: delays, non-disclosure and partial disclosure. What the research tells us and implications for practice. *Child Abuse Review*, 24(3), 159–169. doi:10.1002/car.2280

Mooney, J., & McGregor, C. (2018). How adults tell: messages for society and policy makers regarding disclosures of childhood sexual abuse. Unpublished PhD thesis. School of Political Science and Sociology, National University of Ireland, Galway.

Myerhoff, B. G. (1992). *Remembered Lives: The Work of Ritual, Story Telling and Growing Older*. University of Michigan Press.

Pack, M. (2004). Sexual abuse counsellors' responses to stress and trauma: a social work perspective. *Journal of New Zealand Association of Counsellors, Te Ropu Kaiwhiriwhiri o Aotearoa*, 25(2), 1–17.

Pack, M. (2016). *Self-Help for Trauma Therapists: A Practitioner's Guide*. Routledge.

Pearlman, L. A., & Saakvitne, K. W. (1995). *Trauma and the Therapist: Countertransference and Vicarious Traumatization in Psychotherapy with Incest Survivors*. W. W. Norton.

Rutter, M. (1987). Psychosocial resilience and protective mechanisms. *American Journal of Orthopsychiatry*, 57, 316–331.

Ullman, S. E., Foynes, M. M., & Tang, S. S. S. (2010). Benefits and barriers to disclosing sexual trauma: a contextual approach. *Journal of Trauma and Dissociation*, 11(2), 127–133.

Wahab, S., Rahman, F. N. A., Mohd Hashim, S., & Razali, S. (2013). Intrafamilial sexual abuse in an Asian society: understanding the victim's internal conflicts. *International Medical Journal*, 20(2), 186–187. www.scopus.com/inward/record.uri?eid=2-s2.0-84878281572&partnerID=40&md5=ff493b0a2085e812e9070448bc0453dd

White, M. (1995). *Re-authoring Lives: Interviews and Essays*. Dulwich Centre.

Wilson, D., Moloney, E., Parr, J. M., Aspinall, C., & Slark, J. (2021). Creating an Indigenous Māori-centred model of relational health: a literature review of Māori models of health. *Journal of Clinical Nursing*, 30(23–24), 3539–3555. doi:10.1111/jocn.15859

Wilson, J., & Lindy, J. (Eds.). (1994). *Countertransference in the Treatment of PTSD*. Guilford Press.

Winnicott, D. (1965). *The Maturational Processes and the Facilitating Environment*. Hogarth Press and the Institute of Psychoanalysis.

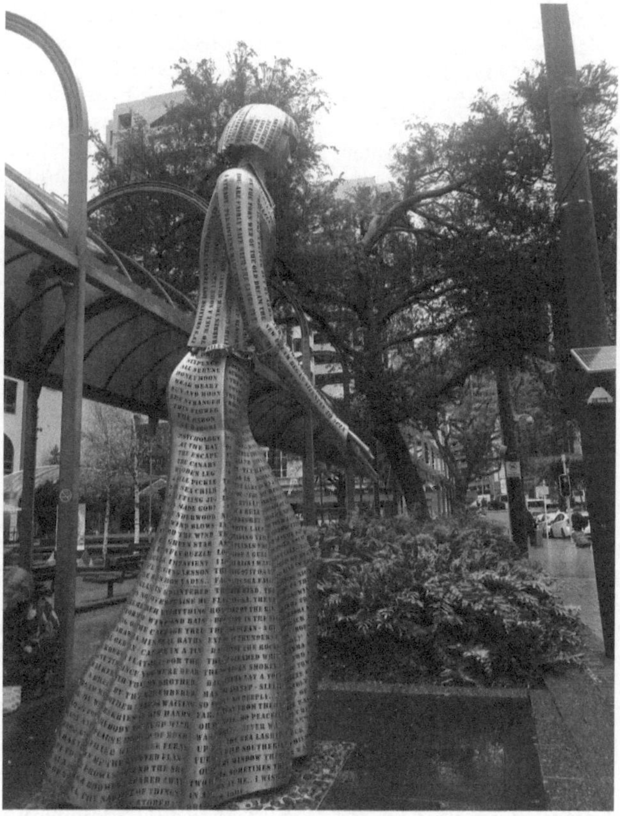

Figure 8.2 'Woman of Words' by renowned sculptor Virginia King

Index